Brief Contents

Part 5: Managing Personal and Practical Issues

Living Well with
HIV & AIDS

2nd Edition

Allen L. Gifford, M.D.

Kate Lorig, R.N., Dr. P.H.

Diana Laurent, M.P.H.

Virginia González, M.P.H.

Bull Publishing Company
Palo Alto, CA

Copyright © 2000 Bull Publishing Company

Bull Publishing Company
P.O. Box 208
Palo Alto, CA 94302-0208
Phone (650) 322-2855   Fax (650) 327-3300
www.bullpub.com

ISBN 0-923521-52-6

Distributed to the trade by:
Publishers Group West
1700 Fourth Street
Berkeley, CA

Publisher: James Bull
Production: Publication Services
Cover Design: Lightbourne Images

Library of Congress Cataloging-in-Publication Data

Living well with HIV & AIDS / Allen L. Gifford . . . [et al.].--2nd ed.
    p. cm
  Includes bibliographical references and index.
    ISBN 0-923521-52-6
    1. AIDS (Disease)--Popular works. I. Title: Living well with HIV and AIDS. II.
Gifford, Allen L.

RC607.A26 L587 2000
362.1'969792--dc21

                                                                00-023029

10 9 8 7 6 5 4 3 2 1

Detailed Contents

PART 2: Managing Your Medical Treatment

Part 5: Managing Personal and Practical Issues

Acknowledgments

This book was produced with the help of many people. First and foremost for acknowledgment are the efforts of the many people with HIV/AIDS, and their friends and families, who have made suggestions about things that should be included in this book and ways to improve it. And many of the ideas included here are from doctors, nurses, health educators, and other health professionals who have devoted themselves to improving the lives of people with HIV/AIDS.

The work represented here would not be possible without the support of the Health Services Research and Development Program and the Quality Enhancement Research Initiative of the U.S. Veterans Health Administration, the National Institute of Nursing Research, the California Universitywide AIDS Research Program, the Office of AIDS Research of the National Institutes of Health, the Lawrence S. Linn Research award, and the Robert Wood Johnson Clinical Scholar Program.

Certain individuals require special mention. Chris Adams helped conceive and plan this project, and his intelligence, wit, and bravery in facing his own illness inspired us all. Special thanks also go to Halsted Holman, Samuel Bozzette, Marian Minor, David Sobel, Vivian Vestal, Janet Tobacman, Joe DiMilia, Jill Bormann, Marty Shively, Sonia Melendez, Lynn Gordon, and all the extraordinary nurses, staff, and physicians who care for people with HIV at the San Diego Veterans Affairs Hospital, the University of California–San Diego, and the University of California–San Francisco.

to Chris Adams

How to Use This Book

No one wants to have HIV or AIDS. But just because you have HIV/AIDS* doesn't mean that life comes to an end. This book has been written to help people with HIV/AIDS learn a healthy way to live. Now this may sound strange. How can one have an illness and live a healthy life at the same time? To answer this question, it is important to think about what "health" really is: *Health is soundness of body and mind, and a healthy life is a life which seeks that soundness.* Therefore, a healthy way to live with any illness is to work at overcoming the physical and emotional problems caused by the illness. The goal is to achieve the greatest possible physical capability and pleasure from life. People with all kinds of illnesses do this successfully every day. That is what this book is all about.

But can people with HIV/AIDS live healthy lives? Of course. HIV/AIDS is a chronic disease like many others. It has many similarities with conditions such as diabetes and heart disease, to name just two. If HIV/AIDS becomes symptomatic, it causes decreased function of the immune system. The chronic symptoms that may result can cause people to lose physical conditioning. In addition, these symptoms may cause feelings of emotional distress, such as depression, frustration, and helplessness. All these things can affect how life is lived. The job of the person living with HIV/AIDS is to find ways to deal with these symptoms and decrease the effects of HIV on life. To do this well, you need to be involved in planning and decision making about how you're going to live with your illness. You need to be a *self-manager*.

You will not find any miracles or cures in these pages. Rather, you will find tips, ideas, and resources about how to become an HIV/AIDS self-manager and make your life better. This advice comes from physicians, health professionals,

---

*The terminology used in discussing HIV-related disease is clumsy. We don't want to just use the term *AIDS* because this word would exclude all the people with HIV infection who don't have an AIDS diagnosis. Therefore, throughout this book we will often use the term *HIV/AIDS* to refer in general to the full range of conditions caused by HIV infection.

psychologists, and, most important, from people like you who have learned to manage living with their HIV/AIDS. Part 1 of the book, HIV/AIDS Self-Management, will introduce you to the concepts and skills you need to become an HIV/AIDS self-manager. Part 2, Managing Your Medical Treatment, provides information about medications and working with your health care team to make treatment decisions. Part 3, Managing Your Symptoms, will help you evaluate and begin to control some of the symptoms you may experience. Part 4, Managing Exercise and Diet, contains information about a healthy approach to exercising and eating. And Part 5, Managing Personal and Practical Issues, will help you approach some important issues of daily living and the losses caused by HIV/AIDS.

HIV/AIDS affects the lives of all kinds of people, with differing personal histories, sexual preferences, and cultural backgrounds. Also, HIV/AIDS affects people if they're HIV-positive without symptoms as well as if they develop symptoms or AIDS illnesses. And the people who *care about* people with HIV/AIDS and live with them and care for them—these people are also affected. This book will be helpful for all these people.

This is not a "textbook"—you don't have to sit down and read every word in every chapter. Instead, read the next two chapters and then use the table of contents to find what you need. Many people pick and choose; feel free to skip around. You may want to start with some background information about HIV/AIDS and its symptoms and treatments. People who don't have symptoms may want to start by learning about exercise, healthy eating, and stress reduction. And people with all stages of HIV can use the knowledge here to help figure out whether a new symptom is a regular "bug" or an urgent condition that needs to be checked out by the doctor. Become familiar with the information in the different sections, and use it in the order that's helpful for you.

This book is not a complete encyclopedia of HIV/AIDS. Information and resources for people with HIV/AIDS are always changing, so while we hope that the "leads" given here will be useful, we want them to just be good starting points. If you have any good tips or helpful hints you want to pass on to others, please write us at the address below. We will incorporate them into future editions of this book.

Please send your ideas or tips to:

Allen L. Gifford, MD
University of California, San Diego
VA San Diego Healthcare System
3350 La Jolla Village Drive 111N-1
San Diego, CA 92161

HIV/AIDS
Self-Management

1   Overview of HIV/AIDS Self-Management

HIV/AIDS is a chronic disease like many others. But what does this mean? To learn to be an HIV/AIDS self-manager, it's important to know how acute and chronic diseases differ and why those differences are important.

Acute and Chronic Conditions

We think of a health problem as being either "acute" or "chronic." Acute health problems usually begin abruptly with a single, easily diagnosed cause; they last for a limited time, and they respond to a specific treatment, such as medication or surgery. For most acute illnesses, a cure with return to normal health is to be expected. For the patient and the doctor, there is relatively little uncertainty. One usually knows what to expect. The illness typically has a cycle of getting worse for a while, being treated, and then getting better. The care of an acute illness depends on a health professional's knowledge and experience to find and administer the correct treatment.

Appendicitis is an example of an acute illness. It typically begins rapidly, signaled by nausea and pain in the abdomen. The diagnosis of appendicitis, established by physical examination, leads to surgery for removal of the inflamed appendix. There follows a period of recovery and then a return to normal health.

Chronic illnesses are different. They begin slowly and proceed slowly. For example, a person with arteriosclerosis ("hardening of the arteries") might have chest pains or breathing problems. Most arthritis starts with little annoying twinges, which gradually increase. Unlike acute disease, chronic illnesses have many causes that vary over time and include heredity, lifestyle factors (smoking, lack of exercise, poor diet, stress, and so on), environmental factors, and physiological factors.

HIV/AIDS is a chronic disease and in many ways is quite similar to other chronic diseases, such as heart disease, stroke, and diabetes. Like these other diseases, HIV/AIDS is sometimes interrupted by acute infections or conditions. For example, a person with HIV may have day-in, day-out chronic symptoms of fatigue and then have a brief, acute episode of *Pneumocystis* pneumonia. Knowing the difference between the acute conditions and the chronic conditions associated with HIV/AIDS is quite important, because the acute conditions are sometimes infections ("opportunistic" infections) that need special treatment.

Chronic symptoms with multiple causes can be frustrating for those of us who want quick answers. It is difficult for the doctor and the patient when immediate answers aren't available. In some cases, even when diagnosis is rapid, such as in the case of a stroke or heart attack, long-term effects may be hard to predict. The lack of a regular or predictable pattern is a major characteristic of most chronic illnesses, and especially HIV/AIDS.

Unlike acute disease, in which full recovery is expected, chronic illness usually leads to persistent loss of physical conditioning. Because chronically ill people can tire easily, they may be unable to accomplish what they once could. They may give up recreational activities, such as walking or going to the gym, or chores like shopping, housework, and yard work. This lack of activity speeds up the process of physical deconditioning. At the same time, the loss of physical activity and uncertainty about the future create a sense of helplessness, a feeling that little or nothing can be done to help the situation. Of course, believing nothing can be done is a guarantee that nothing will be done, which reinforces helplessness and perpetuates the vicious cycle. A big problem of living with HIV/AIDS is dealing

Acute versus Chronic Conditions

	Acute Condition	*Chronic Condition*
Example	*Pneumocystis* pneumonia	Fatigue
Beginning	Rapid	Gradual
Duration	Short	Indefinite
Treatment	Cure common	Cure rare
Role of professional	Select and conduct therapy	Teach and advise
Role of patient	Follow professional's instructions/advice	Active partner of health professionals, responsible for daily management

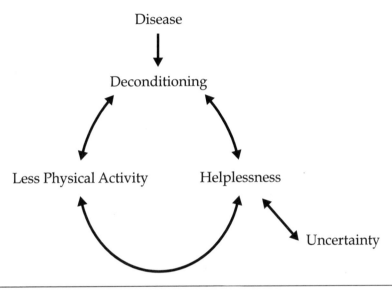

Figure 1.1 The Cycle of Deconditioning

with this cycle of physical deconditioning and helplessness. Throughout this book we examine ways of breaking the cycle and stopping the physical deconditioning and helplessness that have been started by the illness.

Another way in which chronic illness differs from acute illness is that chronic illnesses such as heart disease, diabetes, and HIV/AIDS often have to be treated with medications that need to be taken every day, for life. Using medications properly is a big part of living with HIV/AIDS, and we will discuss medications at length later in the book.

Understanding HIV and AIDS

AIDS is a disease of the immune system caused by a virus—the human immunodeficiency virus, or HIV. People who become infected with HIV develop damage to their immune system gradually over a period of years. When the immune damage is minimal, a person with HIV doesn't notice anything at all. If the immune damage gets worse, the person may notice swollen lymph nodes or get certain mild infections of the skin or mouth. If the immune damage gets quite severe, people with HIV lose the ability to fight off serious infections and cancers that otherwise wouldn't cause much trouble. If one or more of these serious infections or cancers develops, the person is said to have AIDS: Acquired Immune Deficiency Syndrome.

In the next several pages, we will discuss how HIV is (and isn't) transmitted and what HIV does to the immune system. Some readers may find this information frightening, but it's impossible to be a self-manager without knowledge of the basics. Knowing medical details about HIV/AIDS should not lead you to lose track of three vital overall facts:

- HIV/AIDS is treatable. People in treatment are living longer and better now than ever in the past.

- Treatments for HIV/AIDS are improving all the time. People starting treatment now have many more therapy options than ever before.

- Each person with HIV/AIDS has a unique experience. People can give you probabilities, but no one can say what will happen to you. For example, it's a mistake to assume that you will have a side effect to anti-HIV "cocktail" medications just because you know someone who did.

How Do People Catch AIDS?

Since AIDS is really the advanced form of infection with HIV, the real question is, How do people catch HIV infection? HIV infects only humans, and the only way to transmit HIV is for the virus to travel from inside one person who is already infected to the blood stream of another person. Some viruses, such as influenza (flu), concentrate in the lungs, so *coughing* spreads them around. Other viruses, such as chicken pox, concentrate in the skin, so *touching* an infected person can spread the disease. HIV is different; it concentrates in the blood and semen, and there aren't many ways to transfer blood and semen from one person to another.

Nearly all the known cases of HIV infection have been transmitted in one of the following ways:

- sexual contact
- injection with contaminated intravenous (IV) needles
- passage of the virus from mother to unborn child
- transfusions of blood or blood products

Note that you can pass HIV on to someone else even if you are taking HIV medication, and even if your HIV viral load is very low, or undetectable.*

Sexual Contact

For an HIV-positive person to have unprotected sex is risky, but exactly how risky depends on exactly what you do during sex. Unprotected anal intercourse appears to be the most effective way to transmit HIV sexually. When a man with HIV puts his bare penis into another person's anus, the receiving person, whether a man or a woman, is at very high risk for catching HIV. Unprotected vaginal intercourse is also risky, though probably a bit less risky than unprotected anal intercourse, since less cracking and bleeding of the skin occur.

There are two reasons why it is vital to practice safer sex if you are HIV positive:

- *To protect others.* Obviously, you would not want to expose someone else to a serious illness.

- *To protect yourself.* Even if you are already HIV positive, you can be reinfected with new, possibly more dangerous strains of HIV. You could be infected with HIV that is drug resistant. Chances are that you will stay healthier longer if you can avoid reinfection. If you have HIV, you are also at increased risk to get other sexually transmitted diseases—such as syphilis, gonorrhea, and hepatitis—through unsafe sex.

Needles and Syringes

HIV-infected people who use a needle and syringe (the plastic container attached to the needle) for injecting drugs leave a small amount of blood in the needle or syringe after they're done. If the needle or syringe is then used by someone else without being sterilized, the first person's blood can be injected into the next person, causing transfer of the infection.

---

*The HIV viral load is a measurement of how much HIV is in the body. We will discuss the HIV load test later in this book.

Mother to Child

The *placenta* is an organ inside a pregnant woman that allows food and oxygen from the mother to go to the baby inside her. If an HIV-positive woman is pregnant, the HIV in her blood can cross the barrier of the placenta and get into her baby's blood while the child is still in the womb. This kind of HIV transmission seems to happen in about one-third of babies born to HIV-positive mothers. When it does happen, the baby will be born infected with HIV. Women with HIV can take medications while they are pregnant to decrease the chances of HIV transmission into the baby.

HIV can also pass from mother to baby in breast milk, though this means of transmission is probably less common. In places with easy access to safe alternatives to breast milk, most doctors say that women with HIV shouldn't breast-feed their babies. But in poorer countries, breast milk may be the healthiest option, even with the risk of HIV.

Blood Transfusion

Blood transfusions were an important source of HIV transmission until the blood test for HIV became available in 1985. Before 1985, blood banks couldn't tell which of the blood units they received had HIV and were therefore dangerous to give to others. Now the risk of getting HIV from a blood transfusion is extremely low.

Other Possible Ways

Everyone agrees about how risky it is to have unprotected sex or to share dirty hypodermic needles between an HIV-positive person and an HIV-negative person. But certain other activities are harder to be sure about. Kissing deeply with exchange of saliva is a good example. Saliva contains extremely low concentrations of HIV, so infection from saliva seems unlikely. But because of sores, bleeding gums, and bites, blood in the mouth is common and not always easy to detect. In theory, this blood could transmit HIV. In practice, no cases of HIV infection due to kissing have ever been proven.

What Does HIV Infection Do?

People who are infected with HIV experience a slow deterioration of their immune system. The immune system is vital to proper functioning of the human

Ways of Catching HIV from an HIV-Positive Person

Definitely Risky	Low Risk	Not Risky
Unprotected anal sex	Mouth-to-genitals sex*	Shaking hands
Unprotected vaginal sex	Kissing with saliva exchange	Sharing bathroom
Sharing unclean needles	Sharing razor or toothbrush	Touching doorknobs
Mouth-to-anus sex		Casual social contact
		Contact with sweat
		Insects

* Although unprotected oral sex is not as risky as anal or vaginal sex, recent research shows that it definitely can transmit HIV.

body, and that's why people with HIV infection can have so much trouble. The human immune system has many different components: there are infection-fighting white blood cells; there are messenger chemicals that signal parts of the system to turn on and off depending on what invader is causing problems; there are natural human toxins ("killer" chemicals) that can destroy invading organisms; and there are proteins that can "tag" invaders, making them more easily attacked by the rest of the immune system. All of the parts of the immune system are important, but HIV particularly attacks one part of the immune system, a type of white blood cell called *T cells* (also called *T helper, T4*, or *CD4+ cells*). People with HIV/AIDS have problems with certain specific types of infections and cancers—the infections and cancers ordinarily controlled by good T cell function.

HIV can also infect brain cells, cells inside the bones (the bone marrow), and cells in the lining of the intestines. Because of the effect on brain cells, some people develop confusion and memory problems if their condition is quite advanced. Since blood cells are made in the bone marrow, the effect of HIV on the bone marrow can lead to decreased blood count (anemia). Chronic problems with diarrhea may come from the effect of HIV on the intestines.

It used to be that the average time from HIV infection to development of full-blown AIDS was eleven years. This was an estimated average time for everyone with HIV, so some people developed AIDS sooner and some later. Now we have stronger and better medications, so people who take the medications can hope to do very well for many years. No one can predict what will happen to any one individual.

HIV infection can be divided into four stages:

1. primary HIV infection, or acute HIV
2. healthy carrier state
3. early symptomatic HIV infection
4. AIDS

Primary HIV infection is the illness that occurs within two to four weeks after a person has become infected with HIV from another person, either by having sex, or by sharing needles. Not everyone has symptoms from primary HIV infection, but in some people it can cause fever, rash, sore throat, aching muscles, cough, swollen lymph nodes, diarrhea, nausea, and vomiting. In other words, it can be like a very bad flu infection. Primary HIV infection usually lasts only a few weeks, but many experts believe that seeing a doctor and having HIV detected during primary infection is a big help, since this may be a good time to start anti-HIV therapy. After primary infection, a person with HIV goes into a healthy carrier state. During this phase, many people won't know that they have HIV, and they will feel fine—but unfortunately they can transmit HIV to others. People who develop early symptomatic HIV infection will start to experience tiredness, fevers, skin and mouth infections, and blood test abnormalities. AIDS is the most advanced of the four stages of HIV infection. People with AIDS have a lot of damage to their T cells and immune systems. If the damage gets severe enough, HIV-positive people may develop certain infections or cancers. If they do, they are said to have progressed to AIDS.

Illnesses Associated with HIV

Most of the severe problems that come from having HIV are caused by the infections and cancers that occur when the immune system gets weak. Because of new medications for HIV, rates of AIDS infections and cancer have dropped sharply compared with ten years ago. The most common illnesses are discussed next.

Pneumocystis carinii Pneumonia (PCP)

Pneumonia (lung infection) caused by the parasite *Pneumocystis carinii* was once the most common AIDS-related illness in the United States. We're now much better at preventing *Pneumocystis* with anti-HIV and anti-*Pneumocystis* medicines, but PCP is still one of the most common AIDS illnesses. Preventive therapy involves treating people at high risk for getting PCP with low doses of PCP drugs so that they never get the disease. This approach has saved many people.

Candida

Candida is a fungus that is commonly found in the mouth, skin, gastrointestinal tract, and vagina. Candida of the esophagus (the swallowing tube between the mouth and stomach) is the most common AIDS illness in the United States right now. Candida of the mouth (thrush) or vagina is even more common, but isn't considered an AIDS illness. Candida takes the form of white spots or patches that can be easily scraped off with a stick. When candida is in the esophagus, it can make it painful to swallow. For some people, finding thrush is the first sign of problems with the immune system. Antifungal medicines are usually very effective.

Bacterial Pneumonia

Pneumonias caused by common community bacteria are now an important problem for people with HIV. These bacterial pneumonias can be treated with antibiotics if they're caught early, and vaccines can help prevent them. The flu vaccine helps, since catching the flu virus can lead to bacterial pneumonia. And medicines to prevent PCP (such as Septra or Bactrim) also help to prevent bacterial infection.

Kaposi's Sarcoma (KS)

Kaposi's sarcoma is a type of slow-growing skin cancer that initially appears as a purple, brown, or pink bump on the skin. It may be very limited and not cause much trouble, but sometimes it can spread widely on the skin and even spread to the internal organs. KS is seen primarily in gay men; it's rare in heterosexuals, even in IV drug users. When it's mild, KS may not need any treatment. But in severe cases, anticancer drugs (chemotherapy) may be needed.

Toxoplasmosis of the Brain

Toxoplasmosis is caused by a parasite (*Toxoplasma gondii*) found in undercooked meat and is a common infection of humans as well as many animals. *Toxoplasma* is also often found in cat litter boxes, in dirt, and in other places where animals leave their wastes. Because of this, people with HIV/AIDS need to be careful to wear gloves when changing cat litter or working in the garden. Usually "toxo" causes very few problems; for most people the immune system controls the infection without any trouble. But in people with AIDS, the infection tends to go to the brain and cause strength, speech, seizure, or walking problems. Sometimes it can go to the internal organs as well. If it's caught early enough, toxoplasmosis can be controlled by taking oral medicines.

Mycobacterium avium Complex (MAC) or *Mycobacterium avium intracellulare* (MAI)

Mycobacterium avium is a bacterium that can spread widely through the blood and internal organs of people with AIDS. People who have a CD4 cell count of less than 50 cells per microliter should take an antibiotic regularly to *prevent* MAC. Treating MAC once the infection starts is more difficult; it usually requires taking two or three different types of antibiotics for long periods, perhaps indefinitely.

Cytomegalovirus (CMV)

Cytomegalovirus is a very common virus that most people have been exposed to long before they become exposed to HIV. Only when the immune system is weakened does CMV start to cause problems in the eyes, intestinal tract, and sometimes other internal organs. CMV can damage the backs of the eyes (CMV retinitis), causing partial loss of vision and even blindness when it's very severe. In the intestinal tract (CMV colitis or enteritis), CMV causes pain, ulcers, bleeding, and diarrhea. Like MAC, CMV is most commonly seen when the T cell count has dropped below 100. Medications can slow and sometimes even stop the problems caused by CMV, but most of the medications require an IV (intravenous line) in your arm or chest.

Tuberculosis (TB)

TB is found in non-HIV-infected people as well as those with HIV, but people with HIV catch it much more easily and in a more severe form. TB is caused by *Mycobacterium tuberculosis,* a bacterium that mostly infects the lungs. But in some people with AIDS, TB can spread throughout the body. TB is particularly common in people who don't have adequate access to medical care. It causes cough, fever, and weight loss and spreads easily through the air around a person coughing out the TB bacteria. Fortunately, we can identify many people who have been exposed to TB by doing skin tests. People on effective treatment are no longer infectious to others. The treatment needed may be as many as four or more oral medicines, and it usually has to be given for a year or more. But staying on the TB medicine is very important—not only for the person with TB, but to protect other people.

Herpes Infections

There are two main types of herpes viruses, herpes simplex and herpes zoster. Herpes simplex type I causes sores (commonly known as cold sores) on the mouth and lips; herpes simplex type II causes sores on the genitals and anus. Sometimes herpes simplex can spread to other parts of the body. Herpes zoster is caused by the same virus that causes chicken pox. It often causes *shingles*, a painful rash that appears on one section of the skin. Again, in severe cases, herpes zoster can spread. Either type of herpes can affect people who don't have HIV, but it is often one of the early infections experienced by people with HIV. If the infection spreads to the eyes, it can be dangerous to the vision. There are medicines to treat some herpes infections, but others, including zoster, can be difficult to treat.

Cryptosporidiosis

In cryptosporidiosis, a parasite *(Cryptosporidium parvum)* infects the intestines and can cause diarrhea and cramping in the abdomen. The parasite is found in many animals and is passed on when food or water gets contaminated. People with normal immune systems get rid of the parasite quite easily; those with a weakened immune system may never do so. Unfortunately, cryptosporidiosis is very difficult to treat. The most important task is to make sure that people with this disease don't get too dehydrated. Cryptosporidiosis and cryptococcosis are easy to mix up, but they're completely different.

Lymphoma

Lymphoma is a cancer of the lymph system caused by uncontrolled growth of abnormal lymph system cells. The most common lymphoma in people with HIV is a type called non-Hodgkin's lymphoma. It can appear as fever, or night sweats with painless enlargement of a lymph node (gland) in one part of the body, with no growth of the lymph nodes in the other parts of the body. It also can start in the brain and cause headaches, localized weakness, speech problems, or seizures. Non-Hodgkin's lymphoma is very difficult to treat. Chemotherapy is required and will sometimes shrink the tumor, but rarely, if ever, cures it completely.

HIV/AIDS as a Chronic Disease

HIV/AIDS can be similar to other chronic conditions in the sense that damage to the immune system may lead to problems with the lungs, causing the body to be deprived of oxygen, which leads to loss of function. But HIV can also lead to loss of function in other ways. Nerve cell damage caused by the virus can cause numbness or discomfort in the feet and hands. Problems in the intestines may decrease the absorption of fluids and important nutrients. Furthermore, the overall work that the body has to do to fight HIV in the cells can lead to an energy drain and fatigue. These things don't always happen, but if any one of them does, it can lead to pain and disability.

Although all chronic illness starts at the cellular level, one does not always know that a disease is present until the symptoms start (shortness of breath, fatigue, pain, and so on). Illness is more than cellular malfunction. It also includes problems with everyday life, such as not being able to do the things you want to do or needing to change your social activities.

Though the biological causes of chronic diseases differ, the problems they create for patients are similar. For example, most people with chronic disease suffer fatigue and loss of energy. Sleeping problems are not uncommon. Some people may have pain, while others may have trouble breathing. Disability, to some extent, is also part of chronic disease.

Another common problem with HIV/AIDS and other chronic illnesses is depression, or just "feeling blue." It is hard to be cheerful when your condition causes serious health problems. Along with the depression come fear and concern for the future. Will I be able to remain independent? If I can't care for myself, who will care for me? What will happen to my family? Will I get worse? Disability and depression bring loss of self-esteem.

Finally, the management tasks and skills one must learn are about the same for any chronic illness. Besides overcoming the physical and emotional problems, it is important to learn problem-solving skills and ways to respond to the trends in your disease. These tasks and skills include using medications appropriately and minimizing the side effects, developing and maintaining health with appropriate exercise and nutrition, managing symptoms, making decisions about when to seek medical help, working effectively with your doctor, finding and using community resources, talking about your illness with family and friends, and if necessary, changing social interactions. The most important skill of all is learning to respond to your illness on an ongoing basis to solve day-to-day problems as they arise.

In this book, we talk about the skills needed to manage HIV/AIDS as well as how to use the principles that have been successful in managing other chronic illnesses. Before we discuss specific management techniques, however, it is necessary to explain what we mean by self-management.

The Job of Self-Management

The first responsibility of any manager is to understand what is being managed. Initially, this may seem like an impossible task. After all, HIV/AIDS is a very complicated and challenging disease that sometimes stumps the best of specialists. But understanding HIV/AIDS is not as difficult as it might seem, for two reasons. First, as a result of daily living with the consequences of the illness, you and your family will become familiar with the way HIV affects your body and what the treatment does for you. You will also know better than anyone what problems *you* experience with medications and side effects. With experience, you may become better able than health professionals to judge your disease and the effects of your treatment. Second, most chronic illnesses go up and down in intensity; they do not have a steady path. Therefore, being able to identify the ups and downs in the path is essential for good management. These ups and downs can be important in making decisions about medications for pain, breathing problems, nausea, or other symptoms.

For example, the visits illustrated in Figure 1.2 represent Pat's regular follow-up appointments with the doctor. Even though the intensity of Pat's symptoms is the same for all three visits, what has happened between the appointments can make a big difference to the health care team in evaluating whether to change Pat's treatment or keep it the same. In the case of the January visit, the symptoms are getting better, so keeping the treatment the same or even lessening it may be in order. In the case of the February visit, the symptoms seem to be getting worse, so additional treatment may be the choice. In the case of the March visit, things have been stable for a while, so maintaining the treatment may be the best option.

Your experience and understanding of how you are doing are often a more useful indicator to your doctor than laboratory tests or other measures. If the physician encourages your learning and you respond by participating in decisions, a partnership is born. To be most effective, self-management in HIV/AIDS requires such a partnership.

When you develop any chronic illness, you become more aware of your body. Minor symptoms that you used to ignore may now cause great concern. For example, is this cough a signal of pneumonia? Is this pain in my leg a sign that neuropathy (chronic nerve pain) has started? There are no simple, reassuring answers

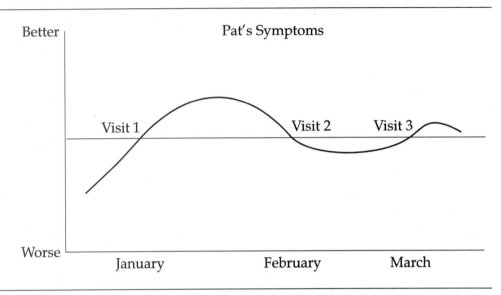

Figure 1.2

to apply to all patients. Nor is there a fail-safe way of sorting out serious signals from minor temporary symptoms that can be ignored. In general, symptoms should be checked out with your doctor if they are *unusual, severe, persistent,* or *occur after starting a new medication.* Some other guidelines are provided in Chapter 7, "Evaluating Common Symptoms of HIV."

Throughout this book, we give some specific examples of what actions to take if you experience certain symptoms. But this is where your partnership with your doctor becomes most critical. He or she can help guide you in responding to specific problems or symptoms. Self-management does not mean going it alone. Get help or advice when you are concerned or uncertain.

Both at home and in the business world, effective managers direct the show, but they don't do everything themselves. They work with others to get the job done. What makes them managers is that *they are responsible* for making the decisions and making sure these decisions are carried out. As a manager of your illness, your job is much the same. You gather information and work with a team of consultants consisting of your physician, other health professionals, and support people such as family and friends. Once they have given you their best advice, it is up to you to follow through. All chronic illness needs day-to-day management. We have all noticed that some people with severe physical problems get on well, whereas others with lesser problems seem to give up on life. The difference is often attitude and management style.

Managing a chronic illness, like managing a family or a business, is a complex undertaking. There are many twists, turns, and midcourse corrections. By learning self-management skills, you can ease the problems of living with your condition.

The keys to success in any undertaking are:

- deciding what you want to do
- deciding how you are going to do it
- learning a set of skills and practicing until you have mastered them

These tasks are all based on your learning skills and mastering them. Success in HIV/AIDS self-management is the same. In fact, mastering such skills is one of the most important tasks of life.

We will describe several skills and strategies to help relieve the problems caused by HIV/AIDS. We do not expect you to use all of them. Pick and choose. Experiment. Set your own goals. What you do may not be as important as the sense of confidence and control you gain by successfully doing something you want to do. However, we have learned that knowing the skills is not enough. You need a way of incorporating these skills into your daily life. In trying a new skill, the first attempts are usually clumsy and slow and show few results. It is easier to return to old ways than to continue trying to master new and sometimes difficult tasks. The best way to master new skills is through practice and evaluation of the results.

Self-Management Skills

What you do about something is largely determined by how you think about it. For example, if you think that having HIV is like running in the dark toward a cliff, not knowing when you will fall over the edge, you might feel no control over what happens and therefore do nothing at all to help yourself. The thoughts you have can greatly determine what happens to you and how you handle your health problems.

The most successful self-managers are people who think of their illness as a path rather than as a cliff. This path, like any path, goes up and down. Sometimes it is flat and smooth. At other times the way is rough. To negotiate this path you have to use many strategies. Sometimes you can go fast; at other times you must slow down. Effective self-managers are people who have learned the skills to negotiate this path.

Self-management skills fall into three main categories:

- *Skills needed to deal with the illness.* Any illness requires that you do new things. These may include taking many medicines and sticking to complicated medication schedules. Sometimes there are new exercises or a new eating plan. Taking care of the illness also means more frequent interaction with your doctor and the health care system. All of these constitute the work you must do to manage your illness.

- *Skills needed to continue your normal life.* Just because you have HIV does not mean that life stops. There are still chores to do, friendships to maintain, jobs to go to, and a multitude of family relationships to carry on. Things that you once took for granted can become much more complicated in the face of HIV/AIDS. You may need to learn new skills in order to maintain your daily activities and to enjoy life.

- *Skills needed to deal with emotions.* When you are diagnosed as having HIV/AIDS, your future changes, and with this come changes in plans and changes in emotions. Many of these emotions are negative. They may include anger ("Why me? It's not fair"), depression ("I can't do anything anymore. What's the use?"), frustration ("No matter what I do, it doesn't make any difference. I can't do what I want to do"), or isolation ("No one understands. No one wants to be around someone who is sick"). Negotiating the path of HIV, then, also means learning skills to work with these negative emotions.

Self-Management Tasks

- *Taking care of your illness* (taking medicine, exercising, going to the doctor, changing diet)
- *Carrying out your normal activities* (household chores, employment, social life, and so on)
- *Managing your emotional changes* (working with changes brought about by your illness, such as anger, uncertainty about the future, changed expectations and goals, and sometimes depression. Changes can also happen in your relationships with family and friends.)

2   Becoming an HIV/AIDS Self-Manager

Like any skill, self-management must be learned and practiced. This chapter will start you on your way. Remember, *you are the manager.*

Like the manager of an organization or household, you must have a management plan:

1. *Decide* what you want to accomplish.
2. *Look for alternative ways* to accomplish this goal.
3. Start making short-term plans by *making an action plan* or agreement with yourself.
4. *Carry out your action plan.*
5. *Check the results.*
6. *Make changes* as needed.
7. Remember to *reward yourself.*

Problems sometimes start with a general uneasiness. You are unhappy but not sure why. Upon closer examination, you find you miss contact with old friends who live far away. With the problem identified, you decide to take a trip to visit your friends. You know what you *want to accomplish.* In the past, you could have driven, but you now find it tiring, so you seek *alternative ways* of travel. Among other things, you consider leaving at noon instead of early in the morning, and making the trip in two days instead of one. You consider asking a friend along to share the driving. There is also a train that goes within twenty miles of your destination, or you might fly (although this is more expensive). You decide to take the train. The trip still seems overwhelming, as there is so much to do to prepare. You decide to write down all the steps necessary to make the trip a reality. These include finding a good time to go, buying a ticket, figuring out how to handle luggage, and thinking about how you can manage your medications and meals when you're away from home.

You start by *making an action plan* or agreement with yourself that this week you will call and find out just how much the railroad can help. You also decide to review your medication schedule and meal plans to make sure you have what you need for the trip. You then *carry out your action plan* by calling the railroad and checking your medication and meal needs.

A week later, you *check the results*. Looking back at all the steps to be accomplished, you find that a single call answered many questions. The railroad is able to accommodate your needs for special meals. However, you are still worried about storing your medications during the trip. You *make a change in your plan* by asking a friend about this, and he suggests a place where you can buy special travel containers for all your medications.

Now you are ready to make a new action plan for accomplishing some of the other tasks necessary to make the trip possible. What once seemed like a dream has become a reality.

Now let's go through these seven steps in detail. They are the backbone of any self-management program.

Deciding What You Want to Accomplish

Deciding what you want to accomplish may be the most difficult part. You must be realistic and very specific. Think of all the things you would like to do. One of our self-managers wanted to climb twenty steps to his friend's home so he could join his friend's family for a holiday meal. Another wanted to gain weight to improve his strength. Still another wanted to be more socially active but felt limited by the need to take an oxygen tank everywhere. In each case, the goal was one that would take several weeks or even months to accomplish. In fact, one of the problems with goals is that they often seem like dreams. They are so far off that we don't even try to accomplish them. We'll tackle this problem next. For now, take a moment to write your goals below. When you have finished, put an asterisk (*) next to the goal you would like to work on first.

Goals

1. _____

2. _____

3. _____

Looking for Alternative Ways of Accomplishing the Goal

Sometimes what keeps us from reaching our goal is a failure to see alternatives. Other times, we reject alternatives without knowing much about them.

There are many ways to reach any specific goal. For example, our self-manager who wanted to climb twenty steps could start off with a slow walking program, start to climb a few steps each day, or look into having the family gathering at a different place. The man who wanted to gain weight could decide to keep a log of his daily calorie intake, talk to his doctor about changing some of his medications, or start an exercise program. The self-manager who wanted more social contact could find out about community college classes or support groups, or could call or write friends.

As you can see, there are many options for reaching each goal. The job here is to list the options and then choose one or two on which you would like to work. Sometimes it is hard to think of all the options yourself. If you are having problems, it is time to use a consultant. Share your goal with family, friends, and health professionals. You can call community organizations such as your local AIDS Foundation or Project Inform.* But rather than asking *what* you should do, ask for *suggestions*. It is always good to have a list of options.

Sometimes people don't consider an option because they assume it doesn't exist or is not workable. Try not to make this kind of assumption without investigating first. One woman we know had lived in the same town all her life and felt that she knew all about the community resources. When she was having problems with her health insurance, a friend from another city suggested contacting an insurance counselor. The woman dismissed this suggestion, however, because she *knew* that this service did not exist in her town. Months later the friend came to visit, called the area social service agencies (listed in the telephone book), and located three insurance counseling services. In short, never assume anything. Assumptions are the major enemies to the self-manager.

Once you have identified your options, write them on the following lines and put an asterisk (*) next to the two or three options on which you would like to work first.

---

*These are just two out of many community and national organizations available to people with HIV/AIDS and their friends and families. There's more information about these resources in Chapter 16.

Options

1. _____
2. _____
3. _____
4. _____
5. _____
6. _____

Making Short-Term Plans: Action Planning

The next step is to turn your options into *short-term plans,* which we will call an action plan. An action plan calls for a specific action or set of actions that you can realistically expect to accomplish within the next week. The action plan should be about something *you* want to do or accomplish. You do not make action plans to please your friends, family, or doctor, but rather to please yourself.

Most of us can do things to make ourselves healthier, but we fail to do them. For example, most people with HIV/AIDS can walk—some just across the room, others for a mile or more. However, few people have a systematic exercise program. An action plan helps you to do the things you know you should do and want to do. Knowing how to make a realistic action plan is an important skill that may well determine the success of your self-management program.

1. First, *decide what you will do* this week. For a step climber, this might be climbing three steps every day for four days. The man trying to gain weight may decide to eat six small meals per day. The action must be something *you* want to do and that you feel you can do realistically, a step on the way to your long-term goal. Make sure that your plans call for a *specific* action or behavior; that is, rather than "relax," you will "listen to the progressive muscle relaxation tapes."

2. Next, *make a specific plan.* This is the most difficult and important part of making an action plan. Deciding what you want to do is

worthless without a plan for doing it. The plan should contain all of the following parts:

- Exactly *what* are you going to do? How far will you walk, how will you eat better, what breathing technique will you practice?

- *How much* will you do? Will you walk around the block, eat at least two fruits per day, practice breathing exercises for fifteen minutes?

- *When* will you do this? Again, this must be specific: before lunch, in the shower, when you come home from work? Connecting a new activity with an old habit is a good way to make sure it gets done. Another trick is to schedule your new activity before an old favorite activity, such as reading the paper or watching a favorite TV program.

- *How often* will you do the activity? This is a bit tricky. We would all like to do things every day. However, we are human, and it is not always possible. It is usually best to plan to do something three or four times a week. If you do more, so much the better. **Please note!!** Taking medications is an exception. This must be done exactly as you and your doctor have agreed. Otherwise you will never know whether the medications can help, and you might put yourself in great danger.

Here are a couple of guidelines for writing your action plan that may help you achieve success:

- *Start where you are, or start slowly.* If you can walk for only one minute, start your walking program with walking one minute once every hour or two, not with walking a mile. If you have never done any exercise, start with a few minutes of warm-up. A total of five or ten minutes is enough. If you want to lose weight, set a goal based on your eating behaviors, such as not eating after dinner.

- *Give yourself some time off* (again with the exception of taking medication). All people have days when they don't feel like doing anything. It is better to say you will do something three times a week instead of every day. That way, if you don't feel like walking one day, you can still meet your action plan.

Parts of an Action Plan

1. Something *you* want to do
2. Reasonable (something you can expect to be able to accomplish that week)
3. Behavior specific
4. Answers the questions:

   What?
   How much?
   When? (Think about your day/week—which days, times?)
   How often?
5. Confidence level of 7 or more (that you will complete the *entire* action plan)

Once you've made your action plan, ask yourself the following question: "On a scale of 0 to 10, with 0 being totally unsure and 10 being totally confident, how confident am I that I can complete this action plan?"

If your answer is 7 or above, yours is probably a realistic action plan. Congratulate yourself—you have done the hard work. If your answer is below 7, then you should look again at your plan. Ask yourself why you're not confident. What problems do you foresee? Then see if you can either solve the problems or change your plan to make yourself more confident of success.

Once you have made an action plan you are happy with, write it down and post it where you will see it every day. Keep track of how you are doing and what problems you encounter. We've included an example of an action plan form at the end of this chapter. You may want to make copies of it to use weekly.

Carrying Out Your Action Plan

If your action plan is well written and realistic, fulfilling it is generally pretty easy. Ask family or friends to check with you on how you are doing. Having to report your progress is good motivation.

Keep track of your daily activities while carrying out your plan. All good managers have lists of what they want to accomplish. Check things off as they are completed. This will give you guidance on how realistic your planning was, and it will also be useful in making future plans. Make daily notes, even of the things you don't understand at the time. Later these notes may help you to see patterns and to solve problems.

For example, our stair-climbing friend never did his climbing. Each day he had a different problem: not enough time, being tired, bad weather, and so on. When he looked back at his notes, he began to realize that the real problem was his fear of getting too short of breath and falling. He then decided to do strengthening and breathing exercises, and to climb the stairs when a friend or neighbor was around.

Checking the Results

At the end of each week, see if you have completed your action plan and if you are any nearer to accomplishing your goal. Are you able to walk farther? Have you gained weight? Are you less fatigued? Taking stock is important. You may not see progress day by day, but you should see a little progress each week. At the end of each week, check on how well you have fulfilled your action plan. If you are having problems, this is the time to problem-solve.

Making Midcourse Changes: Problem Solving

When you are trying to overcome obstacles, your first plan may not always be the most practical plan. If something doesn't work, don't give up. Try something else: modify your short-term plans so that your steps are easier, give yourself more time to accomplish difficult tasks, choose new steps to your goal, or check with your consultants for advice and assistance.

1. The first and most important step is to *identify the problem*. This is usually the most difficult step as well. You may know, for example, that keeping up with your work and social activities is a problem for you, but it will take a little more effort to determine that the real problems are managing medications and fatigue interfering with your activities.

2. Once you have identified the problem, the next step is to *list ideas to solve the problem*. You may be able to come up with a good list yourself, but often calling in help from consultants is beneficial.

Problem-Solving Steps

1. Identify the problem (this is the most difficult and most important step).
2. List ideas to solve the problem.
3. Select one method to try.
4. Assess the results.
5. Substitute another idea if the first didn't work.
6. Utilize other resources (ask friends, family, professionals for ideas if your solutions didn't work).
7. Accept that the problem may not be solvable now.

Consultants can be friends, family, members of your health care team, or community resources.

3. When you have a list of ideas, *pick one to try.* As you try something new, remember that new activities are usually difficult. Be sure to give your potential solution a fair chance before deciding it won't work.

4. After you've given your idea a fair trial, assess the results. Was the idea helpful? If all has gone well, your problem will be solved.

5. If you still have the problem, choose another idea from your list and try again.

6. If a solution still eludes you, *use other resources* (your consultants) to get more ideas.

7. If all of the above steps do not work, you may have to *accept that your problem may not be solvable right now.* This is sometimes hard to do. However, just because a problem is not solvable right now doesn't mean that it won't be solvable later or that other problems can't be solved with this method. Even if your path is blocked, there are probably alternate paths. Don't give up. Keep going.

Rewarding Yourself

The best part of being a good self-manager are the rewards you will receive in accomplishing your goals and in living a fuller and more comfortable life.

The Successful Self-Manager

- Sets goals
- Makes a list of alternatives for reaching a goal
- Makes short-term plans or action plans toward that goal
- Carries out the action plan
- Checks on progress weekly
- Makes midcourse changes as necessary
- Uses rewards for a job well done

However, don't wait until your goal is reached—reward yourself frequently. For example, decide that you won't read the paper until after you exercise. Reading the paper then becomes your reward. One self-manager rewards himself with an ice cream cone after finishing each of his medical appointments. Another self-manager who stopped smoking used the money he would have spent on cigarettes to have his house professionally cleaned, and there was even enough left over to go to a baseball game with a friend. Rewards don't have to be fancy, expensive, or unhealthy. There are many healthy pleasures that can add enjoyment to your life.

One last note: Not all goals are achievable. Chronic illness may mean having to give up some options. If this is true for you, don't dwell too much on what you can't do. Rather, start working on another goal you would like to accomplish. One self-manager we know who uses a wheelchair talks about the 90 percent of things he *can* do. He spends his life developing this 90 percent to the fullest.

Now that you understand the meaning of self-management, you are ready to begin using the tools that will make you a self-manager. In Chapters 3 through 6, we talk about medications and their uses. Chapters 7 and 8 contain information on some of the common chronic symptoms with HIV. The rest of the book is devoted to tools of the trade. These include exercise, nutrition, symptom management, communication, making decisions about the future, finding resources, and information about advance directives.

Action Plan Form

In writing your action plan, be sure it includes:

- *What* you are going to do
- *How much* you are going to do
- *When* you are going to do it
- *How many* days a week you are going to do it

For example: This week, I will walk (*what*) around the block (*how much*) before lunch (*when*) three times (*how many*).

This week I will _____ (*what*)

_____ (*how much*)

_____ (*when*)

_____ (*how many*)

How confident are you that you can complete this action plan? _____

(Write a number between 0 and 10, where 0 = not at all confident and 10 = totally confident.)

	Check off	Comments
Monday		
Tuesday		
Wednesday		
Thursday		
Friday		
Saturday		
Sunday		

Managing Your Medical Treatment

3

The Role of Medications

Having HIV/AIDS usually means taking medications. Thus a very important self-management task is to understand your medications and use them appropriately.

Nearly everyone who is getting care for HIV or AIDS has heard of the "cocktail" medications that are available now to treat HIV. These anti-HIV (or *antiretroviral*) drugs are powerful, especially when given in combinations (known as "*highly active antiretroviral therapy*," or HAART). In many people the medications can reduce HIV in the blood so much that it can't be detected by blood tests. People who had been very sick are returning to active, healthy lives. And others can take the medications to keep from getting sick in the first place.

That's the good part. The hard part is that the cocktail drugs do not work well for everyone, and taking HIV medications can be very difficult. This part of the book will discuss some of the basic information you'll need in order to manage your medications for HIV.

A Few General Words about Medications

Almost nothing receives as much advertising as medications. When we read a magazine, listen to the radio, or watch TV, we are bombarded with a constant stream of ads aimed at convincing us that if we just use this pill or potion, our symptoms will be cured. "Recommended by 90 percent of the doctors asked." "Take an aspirin for your headache." Almost as a backlash to this advertising, we have been taught to avoid excess medications. We have all heard about or experienced some of the ill effects of medications. "Just say no to drugs." "Drugs can kill." It is all very confusing.

31

Even so, medications are a very important part of managing HIV/AIDS. So far, medications cannot completely cure the disease, but they can do many things to help people live well:

- Medications that fight HIV directly (such as the cocktail medications) can *slow the disease process*. For example, drug combinations such as indinavir (Crixivan), lamivudine (3TC, Epivir), and zidovudine (AZT, Retrovir) can reduce the effects of HIV and improve the immune system.

- Medications can help *prevent problems from starting*. For example, people at high risk for *Pneumocystis* pneumonia can take medicines to keep from ever getting the pneumonia.

- Medications can *reduce symptoms* through their chemical actions. For example, pain medications decrease activity in nerve cells, which can decrease pain sensations. Nausea medications decrease stomach hyperactivity, quieting stomach upset.

- Finally, there are medications that *replace substances that the body is no longer producing adequately*. Hormones such as testosterone and estrogen are medications of this type.

In all cases, the purpose of medication is to lessen the consequences of disease or to slow its course. However, as you can see, many of the drugs we use will not have a positive effect that you can detect when you take them. Sometimes the drug will stabilize a condition that without the drug would have gotten worse. Sometimes the drug may only slow down a deterioration that would have been more rapid without the drug. It can be easy to think that the drug isn't doing anything. But except for drugs that are taken *just* for symptoms, it's hard to judge just by how you feel whether medications are working or not. That's why it's important to talk openly with your doctor about your medications and discuss any changes you might want to make. This is especially true with anti-HIV HAART medications. If you stop taking some of them, or if you skip doses, you may make the HIV in your body resistant, so that it gets stronger rather than weaker.

HAART medications get the most attention of the medications used by people with HIV. There is so much information about these medications, and so many details to think about, that it's sometimes hard to follow the big picture. These medicines have transformed HIV care, and they are very effective for many people. They may be effective for you—but they also require a big commitment. Taking them is work, and they can lead to side effects or drug resistance if not taken correctly. On the other hand, the benefits are real: people who take the medications are much less likely to get AIDS-related infections and are much less likely to die. Many of them feel a lot stronger and healthier, too.

People who do well on HAART medications are those who understand that they won't always be easy to take but decide to take them anyway.

In addition to being helpful, all medications have side effects. Some are predictable and minor, and some are unexpected and life threatening. Five to 10 percent of all hospital admissions are due to drug reactions. In spite of this, there's no reason to be frightened of medications. By knowing what medications you're using and by knowing what (and what not) to expect, you can maximize your benefit and reduce the chances of serious side effects.

What Is a Side Effect?

A side effect is any effect other than the one you want. Usually, it is an undesirable effect. Examples of undesirable side effects are stomach problems, constipation, diarrhea, sleepiness, and dizziness. You should know the common side effects of the medications you take. Sometimes people say they can't or won't take a drug because of its possible side effects. This is understandable. However, before you make a decision to stop taking a drug or refuse to take it, you should ask yourself and your doctor the following questions.

Are the benefits from this medication more important than the side effects?

HIV cocktail drugs are a good example of medications whose benefits should be weighed against their undesirable side effects. Although these drugs have side effects, many people still choose them because of their life-saving qualities. To start or not start the drugs is your decision. However, you should always ask yourself, "Will I be better off with the drug despite the side effects?"

Are there ways of avoiding the side effects or making them less severe?

Many times the way you take the drug—for example, with or without food—can make a difference. Ask your doctor or pharmacist for advice on this question.

Are there other medications that have the same benefits but fewer side effects?

Sometimes various drugs can do the same thing but react differently in different people. Unfortunately, you cannot know how you will react to a drug until you have taken it. Therefore, your doctor may have to try different medications before hitting on the ones that are best for you.

The effects and side effects of HIV medications can be very complicated, and it can be tough to figure out how to minimize the side effects and still get the benefits you need. Your doctor, nurse, and pharmacist are your main resources for advice about your medications, and you need to talk to them whenever you think of making a change. But there are lots of places to get helpful information. Some information about medications and side effects is included later in this book. We've also listed sources of information about HIV medications at the end of this chapter and in Chapter 16.

Monitoring the Effects of Medication on HIV

People with HIV may get lots of different blood tests, but two tests are particularly important for monitoring how active HIV is in your body and how much your immune system is affected. The first is the *viral load* test, also called the HIV plasma RNA test or the PCR test. The second is the *T cell* or *CD4+ cell* test. It is important that you know the basics of both of these tests in order to understand and consider treatments for HIV.

Viral Load Test

The virus is constantly multiplying in a person with HIV, but whether it multiplies quickly or slowly depends on the immune system and on the medications being used. Measuring the level of HIV in the blood is a way of telling how active the HIV infection is. The more HIV in the blood, the more the virus can damage the immune system. People with a high level of HIV activity in their blood (high viral load) are generally advised to take a combination of anti-HIV medications. People with very low HIV activity in their blood (low viral load) may be advised to wait.

There are different tests to measure HIV in the blood, but they all count the number of HIV particles (HIV RNA) in the blood. The RT-PCR (reverse-transcriptase polymerase chain reaction) test and the bDNA (branched-chain

DNA) test are the two most common. Measurements are usually reported as the number of virus copies (that is, HIV RNA) in each milliliter of blood. The virus may be "undetectable" (fewer than 20–400 copies, depending on the specific test), it may be detectable but low (fewer than 10,000 or 20,000 copies per milliliter), or it may be quite high (over a million copies). Because the numbers range so widely, a tenfold or even a hundredfold drop in viral levels is possible with effective treatment. This means that someone with 100,000 HIV copies per milliliter before treatment could drop to 1000 copies per milliliter.

T Cell or CD4+ Cell Count

Whereas the viral load test tells how active the virus is, the T cell count is the most useful test available for monitoring how much HIV affects the immune system.

The T cell count is simply a blood test that measures the number of T helper cells (or CD4+ cells) in each microliter of blood. Because T cells are important in fighting infections and cancers, having a low T cell count increases the risk of illness. But T cell counts fluctuate quite a bit, even in healthy, HIV-negative people. All kinds of things affect the T cell count, such as stress, sleep, time of day, the lab where the test was done, and the presence of other infections. The T cell count is a bit like your blood pressure: it's important, but it goes up and down, and the trend is more important than any one reading.

Generally speaking, a T cell count between 500 and 1800 is normal for adults. A count between 200 and 500 indicates that the immune system is suppressed, but people in this range are usually not at high risk for getting seriously ill. AIDS-associated diseases are rarely associated with a T cell count over 200. Kaposi's sarcoma (KS), tuberculosis (TB), and lymphoma are exceptions, but when a person's T cell count is over 200, these diseases appear in less dangerous forms. Problems such as oral candida (thrush) and skin problems can appear at this stage.

A T cell count between 50 and 200 indicates that the immune system is severely suppressed. Because of this, one of the criteria of AIDS is any HIV-positive person who has had a T cell count less than 200. Many opportunistic infections (infections that develop when the immune system is weak but not when it's strong) develop when T cells are in this range. People with counts in this range definitely should take medication to prevent *Pneumocystis carinii* pneumonia (PCP). Nevertheless, lots of people with a T cell count less than 200 still feel healthy and have no symptoms.

A T cell count below 50 indicates that the T cell part of the immune system is not functioning. Good, comprehensive medical care is vital, and treatment with medicines to prevent opportunistic infections is very important. Most people who die of AIDS have a T cell count below 50. However, even at this low count, some people will feel well and have no AIDS-related problems. So T cells are important, but they're not the whole story.

Both the viral load and the T cell count must be considered in order to monitor how an individual person is doing. Of course, it's always best to have a high T cell count and a low (or undetectable) viral load. But people with low T cell counts can still do quite well if the viral load is low, indicating that no further weakening of the immune system is taking place. Researchers have developed charts that show how likely it is that a person with HIV will become sick with AIDS, based on viral load and T cell count. This kind of information is important to consider when making decisions about HIV treatment.

What Medications Are Available?

The main treatments used for HIV and AIDS are medications that act in one of four ways:

- *Antivirals* fight the HIV itself by preventing the virus inside the body from reproducing. Protease inhibitors, reverse-transcriptase inhibitors, and all the other "cocktail " drugs work in this way.

- *Preventive medicines* prevent specific opportunistic infections. People with HIV are carefully monitored to find out when they are at high risk for certain specific diseases. Then, if they move into a high-risk group, they can start taking preventive medicines. Preventive strategies for *Pneumocystis*, tuberculosis, toxoplasmosis, and *Mycobacterium avium* complex (MAC) are well established.

- *Treatment medicines* are used to treat specific opportunistic infections and diseases once they are identified.

- *Immune boosters* increase the body's immune response to invaders and to HIV itself. This approach may be promising for the future, but presently it is still experimental, and there are no approved treatments of this type. The therapeutic vaccines being developed fall in this category. We will not give specific examples of medicines in this category, since all are experimental and there is not much reliable information about them. But some researchers think that immune boosters will be necessary if we hope someday to completely cure people with HIV.

In the following pages, we will discuss some of the more common medications used in HIV care. Much more extensive descriptions are widely available (see "Suggested Reading" at the end of this chapter).

Antiviral Medications

The number of antiviral (also called *antiretroviral*) HIV drugs available is growing every year, and while there once were only a few different medication combinations people could use, now there are hundreds. Guidelines for treating HIV all recommend that anti-HIV drugs be used in combinations, usually consisting of at least three drugs. The one exception is women with HIV who are taking medication to prevent the HIV from passing to their babies. In some situations, these women may be treated with zidovudine (AZT) alone. Since antiretrovirals are so important in treating HIV, we will discuss them separately in Chapter 6.

Preventive Medications

Even with good anti-HIV medications available, specific antibiotics continue to play a crucial role in preventing opportunistic infections (see pp. 10–13). Next we list some of the major opportunistic infections, along with descriptions of the medicines used to prevent them.

Pneumocystis carinii Pneumonia (PCP)

Examples: Trimethoprim/sulfamethoxazole (Bactrim, Septra, TMP/SMX),* aerosolized pentamidine (NebuPent, AeroPent), and dapsone. Atovaquone (Mepron) may be an appropriate preventive medication for a few people.

---

*Generic drug names are listed first, with alternate names for each drug in parentheses.

How they work: These medications all work by giving a steady low dose of antibiotic to kill *Pneumocystis* before there are enough organisms to create a true pneumonia.

Possible side effects: With TMP/SMX, the most common side effect is an allergic skin reaction resulting in rashes, which can be successfully managed. Fair-skinned people on TMP/SMX are also sensitive to sunlight. Other side effects include minor fevers, nausea, white count suppression, decreased platelet count, and liver irritation. Dapsone is associated with less severe occurrences of nausea, vomiting, rashes, lowered red and white cell counts, and liver function problems. People with low levels of G6PD (a liver function indicator) can develop rapid loss of blood cells on dapsone, so a G6PD test should be done before beginning dapsone treatment. The most common side effect of aerosolized pentamidine is a cough or raspy, dry throat, which can be minimized or eliminated by the use of inhaled medicines such as albuterol. Other side effects include a burning sensation in the back of the throat, an unpleasant taste, brief lung spasms, and (rarely) a mild decrease in blood sugar. Atovaquone has fewer side effects, but it is also expensive.

Comments: TMP/SMX works extremely well for preventing PCP; almost no one who takes it regularly (daily or three times per week) comes down with the disease. The problem is that many people experience toxic reactions to TMP/SMX. These people may be able to take the medication if they take a gradually increasing dose. Otherwise, they should use one of the other medications.

Toxoplasmosis (Toxo)

Examples: Trimethoprim/sulfamethoxazole (Bactrim, Septra, TMP/SMX), dapsone, clindamycin, atovaquone (Mepron), and pyrimethamine are all used for prevention of toxoplasmosis.

How they work: As with *Pneumocystis,* the idea is to kill the *Toxoplasma* organisms when they are present at microscopic levels, before they have started to invade brain tissue. The medications all work by giving a steady low dose of antibiotic. Steady low doses are particularly important for people with a low CD4 cell count and with a positive blood *Toxoplasma* antibody test.

Possible side effects: The side effects of TMP/SMX and dapsone are the same whether these drugs are used for toxoplasmosis or *Pneumocystis* prevention. Atovaquone has fewer side effects. Clindamycin causes rash and/or diarrhea in many people. Pyrimethamine can cause loss of red blood cells in some people but is well tolerated in most.

Comments: People who need toxoplasmosis prevention almost always need *Pneumocystis* prevention too, so taking either TMP/SMX or dapsone can accomplish both goals. The other medications are less well proven but can be considered for a person who is taking aerosolized pentamidine to prevent *Pneumocystis* and therefore needs another medicine to prevent toxoplasmosis.

Tuberculosis (TB)

Examples: Isoniazid (INH) is the most common medicine for preventing TB in people who have a positive skin test. Rifampin and pyrazinamide may also be used. Still other drugs may be used if the doctor thinks you have been exposed to a resistant form of TB.

How they work: If you're around someone with TB, a small number of organisms may get into your lungs and create a tiny infection. This is enough to make your immune system react and make your skin test positive. INH, given for a year, can kill the infection before it becomes active.

Possible side effects: INH can occasionally cause liver disease. It can also cause neuropathy (nerve damage in the arms and legs), but this is easy to prevent by taking vitamin B6 while you're on the INH.

Comments: The skin test for TB is very important in detecting TB before it becomes active. There is a big difference between taking one medication to prevent TB and waiting until the TB has spread, when usually at least four medications are needed.

Mycobacterium avium Complex (MAC)

Examples: Clarithromycin and azithromycin are effective for preventing MAC, and rifabutin is also sometimes used.

How they work: MAC is different from TB. There is no blood or skin test that can "catch" MAC when you've been exposed but are not yet actively infected. But we do know that the risk of MAC goes up sharply when the T cell count is below 100, and the risk is even higher when the count is below 50. If a person has a low T cell count, taking clarithromycin or azithromycin can reduce the chances of getting MAC. These medicines work by killing the MAC before it can get a "foothold" in the body.

Possible side effects: Clarithromycin and azithromycin can cause stomach upset or diarrhea, but generally they are well tolerated. Rifabutin may cause rashes, stomach upset, or a drop in the white blood cell count.

Cytomegalovirus (CMV)

Examples: Only one medication, oral ganciclovir (Cytovene) is available for *preventing* CMV eye disease. Medicines to treat active CMV disease in the eyes or GI system (ganciclovir, foscarnet) must be given by vein (IV) or by central line (a special IV put in by the doctor that goes directly into the chest). CMV eye disease can also be treated with tiny implants of drug into the eye.

How they work: People at risk for CMV eye disease usually have been exposed to CMV before contracting HIV. Oral ganciclovir works by "holding down" the spread of CMV to the eyes.

Possible side effects: Probably the biggest issue is that people on oral ganciclovir take 12 pills (!) per day, in addition to all the other medications they might be on. For many, this just seems like too much. Not surprisingly, some people have nausea and diarrhea. Ganciclovir can also cause decreased blood cell levels.

Comments: Using oral ganciclovir to prevent CMV retinitis is not a standard practice, but it is something to be considered.

Treatment Medications

Many of the medications just listed for *preventing* problems seen in HIV/AIDS are also used for *treating* the problems when they occur. But treatment is always more difficult; it requires higher doses, more medicines, and more complicated combinations, and it has more side effects. Many, many medications are used for treating different acute infections, so we will not discuss all of them here. Generally speaking, all exert their toxic effects to kill the invading virus, bacteria, parasite, or fungus, and all attempt to do this with minimal toxicity to the cells of the human body. Your treatment team should be your first source for information about medicines used to treat acute infections, but there are also other resources you can use. See the lists that follow.

Suggested Reading

Kearney, Brian, and Petrow, Steven (eds.). *The HIV Drug Book.* New York: Pocket Books, 1998. (An excellent and comprehensive HIV drug reference.)

Ward, Darrell E. *The AmFAR AIDS Handbook.* New York: W.W. Norton & Company, 1999.

Resources

HIV/AIDS Treatment Information

Telephone Information

Centers for Disease Control (CDC) HIV/AIDS Treatment Information Service	(800) 448-0440
National Institutes of Health (NIH) AIDS Clinical Trials Information Service	(800) TRIALS-A
Project Inform Treatment Hotline	(800) 822-7422

World Wide Web Resources

(These change all the time, but are good places to start.)

Center for AIDS Prevention Studies	(http://chanane.ucsf.edu/capsweb/)
Project Inform	(http://www.projectinform.org)
HIVInSite	(http://HIVinsite.ucsf.edu/medical)
AIDS Treatment Information Service	(http://www.HIVatis.org/druginfo.html)

4   Working with Your Doctor

With all the new tests, medications, and research coming out, it might seem that HIV care is impossibly complicated, and that patients should just go to the doctor, listen, and do as the doctor says. However, that's not the way chronic diseases work. Patients with chronic diseases spend very little time with their health care providers. They act as their own "first-line" caregivers—taking medications on their own, and monitoring their daily activities and symptoms on their own or with family members. No matter how complicated or technical your HIV treatment is, no one knows better than you what problems are arising on a day-to-day basis and how the care plan fits into your routine.

People with chronic HIV take care of themselves, with the help of their doctors, nurses, and other experts. So to live well with HIV you need to be able to *work with* your doctor; that means being able to choose a doctor and to talk with him or her about your treatments and about how you're doing. That's what this chapter is about.

Choosing a Doctor

Finding the right doctor is a concern for most people, and even more so for the person with HIV. There are many different kinds of doctors out there, and sometimes it is difficult to know which type of doctor is right for you. While you may need to work with a specialist from time to time for specific problems, a specialist is not always necessary for treating HIV/AIDS. It is best to find a doctor who can help you with all of your health needs. Usually, this is an *internist* for adults and a *pediatrician* for children.

An internist has had special training in the care of adults and can care for most common adult health problems. A pediatrician has had special training in the care of children. Not all internists, pediatricians, or even different specialists, however, are experienced in treating HIV/AIDS. For this reason, when choosing your doctor, look for one who has this experience, preferably one who has many HIV patients as part of his or her practice.

Another factor to consider when choosing your doctor is that he or she be someone you like and can get along with. The sooner you can find such a doctor, the sooner you can begin to build a partnership and develop the best treatment plan for your condition. Being able to establish and maintain this relationship, though, means learning effective ways to communicate with your doctor, especially given the time constraints with which both of you must work during your visits.

Communicating with Your Doctor

The relationship you have with your doctor must be looked on as a long-term one requiring regular work, much like a close partnership. Your doctor will probably know more intimate details about you than anyone except perhaps your spouse, partner, or parents. You, in turn, should feel comfortable expressing your fears, asking questions that you may think are "stupid," and negotiating a treatment plan to satisfy both you and your doctor without feeling "put down" or that your doctor is not interested.

In this partnership between you and your doctor, *the biggest threat to a good relationship and good communication is time.* If you or your doctor were to fantasize about the best thing to happen in your relationship, it would probably involve more time for you both—more time to discuss things, more time to explain things, more time to explore options. When time is short, the resulting anxiety can lead to rushed messages—often "you" messages, and messages that are just plain misunderstood—with no time to correct them.

A doctor is usually on a very tight schedule. This fact becomes painfully obvious when you have to wait in the doctor's office because an emergency has arisen at some time between appointments. Doctors try to stay on schedule, and sometimes patients and doctors alike feel rushed as a consequence. One way to help you to get the most from your visit with the doctor is to take **PART:** Prepare, Ask, Repeat, Take action.

Prepare

Before visiting or calling your doctor, *prepare your "agenda."* What are the reasons for your visit? What do you expect from your doctor? Take some time to make a written list of your concerns or questions. But be realistic. If you have thirteen different problems, it isn't likely that your doctor can adequately deal with that many concerns in one visit. Identify your *main* concerns or problems. Writing them down helps you remember them. Have you ever thought to yourself, after you walked out of the doctor's office, "Why didn't I ask about . . ." or "I forgot to mention . . . ." Making a list beforehand helps to ensure that your main concerns get addressed.

Preparing will also help you to do several important things *during* the visit.

- *Mention your main concerns right at the beginning of the visit.* Give your list to the doctor, and let him or her know which items are the most important to you. If the list is long, expect only two or three items to be addressed in this visit. Studies show that doctors allow an average of eighteen seconds for the patient to state his or her concerns before interrupting with focused questioning. Preparing your questions in advance will help you use your eighteen seconds well. Remember to check your list before you leave to make sure your most important concerns have been addressed.

  Here's an example of how to bring up your major concerns at the beginning of the visit. When the doctor asks, "What brings you in today?" you might say something like "I have a lot of things I want to discuss this visit" *(the doctor immediately begins to feel anxious because of an already overfilled appointment schedule)*, "but I know that we have a limited amount of time. The things that most concern me are my dizziness and the side effects from one of the medications I'm taking" *(the doctor feels relieved because the concerns are focused and potentially manageable within the appointment time).*

- *Describe your symptoms concisely.* This includes when they started; how long they last; where they are located; what makes them better or worse; whether you have had similar problems before; whether you have changed your diet, exercise, or medications in a way that might contribute to the symptoms; and so on. If a treatment has been tried, you should be prepared to report the effect of the treatment. And if you have previous records or test results that might be relevant to your problems, bring them along.

- *Be as open as you can in sharing your thoughts, feelings, and fears.* Remember, your physician is not a mind reader. If you are worried, try to explain *why:* "I am afraid that what I have may be contagious" or "I'm worried the virus has become resistant." The more open you are, the more likely it is that your doctor can help you.

- *Give your physician feedback.* If you don't like the way you have been treated by the doctor or someone else on the health care team, let your doctor know. If you were unable to follow the physician's advice or had problems with a treatment, tell your physician so that adjustments can be made. Also, most physicians appreciate compliments, but patients are often hesitant to praise their doctors. If you are pleased, remember to let your physician know this, too.

Ask

Another key to effective doctor-patient communication is asking questions. Getting understandable answers and information is one of the cornerstones of self-management.

You need to be prepared to ask questions about diagnosis, tests, treatments, and follow-up.

- *Diagnosis.* Ask your doctor what's wrong, what caused it, if it is contagious, what the future outlook (or prognosis) is, and what can be done to prevent it in the future.
- *Tests.* Ask your doctor if more medical tests are necessary, how they will affect your treatment, how accurate they are, and what is likely to happen if you are not tested. If you decide to have a test, find out how to prepare for the test and what it will be like.
- *Treatments.* Ask about your treatment options, including different kinds of medication options. Inquire about the risks and benefits of treatment and the consequences of not treating.
- *Follow-up.* Find out if and when you should call or return for a follow-up visit. What symptoms should you watch for, and what should you do if they occur?

You may want to take some notes during the visit or consider bringing along someone to act as a second listener. Another set of eyes and ears may help you recall some of the details of the visit or instruction later.

Repeat

It is extremely helpful to briefly repeat back to the doctor some of the key points from the visit and discussion, such as diagnosis, prognosis, next steps, and treatment actions. This allows you to double-check that you clearly understood the most important information. It also gives the doctor a chance to quickly correct any misunderstandings and miscommunications. If you don't understand or remember something the physician said, admit that you need to go over it again. For example, you might say, "I'm pretty sure you told me some of this before, but I'm still confused about it." Don't be afraid to ask what you may think is a "stupid" question. Such questions can often bring out an important concern or misunderstanding.

Take Action

When the visit is ending, make sure you clearly understand what to do next. When appropriate, ask your physician to write down instructions or recommend reading material for more information on a particular subject.

If, for some reason, you can't or won't follow the doctor's advice, let the doctor know. Be honest, even if you're worried that what you're saying isn't what the doctor wants to hear—for example, "I can't take the Viracept. It gives me stomach problems, and I always miss the dose in the middle of the day," or "My insurance doesn't cover that, so I can't afford it," or "I've tried to quit smoking before, but everyone I know smokes, and I just can't stay off cigarettes." If your doctor knows why you can't or won't follow the advice, he or she can sometimes make suggestions to help you overcome the barrier. If you aren't open about the barriers to taking action, it's difficult for your doctor to help.

Talking to Your Doctor about Medications

It is common for people with HIV to be taking lots of medications: anti-HIV "cocktail" medications, anti-inflammatory drugs for pain or fever, a pill for depression, an antibiotic to prevent *Pneumocystis*, antacids for heartburn, a tranquilizer for anxiety, plus a handful of over-the-counter (OTC) remedies. *Remember, the more medications you are taking, the greater the risk of drug reactions.* Fortunately, you can often reduce the number of medications and the associated risks if you have forged an effective partnership with your doctor. Such a relationship requires your participation in determining the need for the medication, selecting the medication, properly using the medication, and reporting back to your doctor the effect of the medication.

An individual's response to a particular medication varies depending upon age, metabolism, activity level, and the waxing and waning of symptoms caused by most HIV diseases. Many medications are prescribed on an as-needed ("PRN") basis, so you need to know when to begin and end treatment and how much medication to take. You need to work out a plan with your doctor to suit your individual needs.

For most medications, *your doctor depends on you* to report what effect, if any, the drug has on your symptoms and what side effects you may be experiencing. On the basis of that information, your doctor may continue, increase, discontinue, or otherwise change your medications. A good doctor-patient partnership requires a continuing flow of information. There are important things you need to let your doctor know and critical information you need to receive in return.

Unfortunately, this vital interchange is too often short-changed. Studies indicate that less than 5 percent of patients receiving new prescriptions ask any questions of their physicians or pharmacists. Doctors tend to interpret patient silence as understanding and satisfaction with the information received. Mishaps often occur because patients either do not receive adequate information about medications and don't understand how to take them, or fail to follow instructions given to them. Safe, effective drug use depends on your understanding of the proper use, the risks, and the necessary precautions associated with each medication you take. *You must ask questions.*

The goal of treatment is to maximize the benefits and minimize the risks. Whether the medications you take are helpful or harmful often depends on how much you know about your medications and how well you communicate with your doctor.

What You Need to Tell Your Doctor

Even if your doctor doesn't ask, there is certain vital information you should mention to him or her.

Are you taking any medications?

Report to your physician and dentist *all* the prescription and nonprescription medications you are taking, including experimental medicines, herbs, birth control pills, vitamins, aspirin, antacids, and laxatives. This information is especially important if you are seeing more than one physician because each one may not know what the others have prescribed. Knowing all the medications you are taking is essential for correct diagnosis and treatment. For example, symptoms such as nausea, diarrhea, sleeplessness, drowsiness, dizziness, memory loss, impotence, and fatigue may be due to a drug side effect rather than a disease.

It is critical for your doctor to know what medications you are taking to help prevent problems from drug interactions. Carry an up-to-date list with you, or at least know the names and dosages of all the medications you are taking. Saying that you are taking "the little green pills" usually doesn't help identify the medication. Everyone should get into the habit of doing a "brown bag" medicine check at least once every six months. The idea is simple: put all the medicines you're taking into a bag, and bring them with you when you see your doctor. Review *all* the medicines with your doctor, and make sure you know which to continue and which to stop or discard. Don't forget the over-the-counter and the "as-needed" medications!

Have you had allergic or unusual reactions to any medications?

Describe any symptoms or unusual reactions you have had to medications taken in the past. Be specific: which medication and exactly what type of reaction. A rash, fever, or wheezing that develops after you take a medication is often a true allergic reaction. If any of these symptoms develops, call your doctor at once. Nausea, ringing in the ears, lightheadedness, and agitation are likely to be side effects rather than signs of true drug allergies.

Do you have any major chronic diseases or medical conditions other than HIV?

Many diseases can interfere with the action of a drug or increase the risk of using certain medications. Diseases involving the kidneys or liver are especially important to mention, since these diseases can slow the metabolism of many drugs and increase toxic effects. Your doctor may also have you avoid certain medications if you have or have had such diseases as hypertension, peptic ulcer disease, asthma, heart disease, diabetes, or prostate problems. Be sure to let your doctor know if you could be pregnant or are breast-feeding, since many drugs are not safe to use in those situations.

What medications were tried in the past to treat your disease?

If you have a chronic symptom or symptoms, it is a good idea to keep your own written record of what medications you have taken for the condition and what the effects were. Knowing your past responses to various medications will help guide the doctor's recommendation of any new medications.

However, just because a medication did not work well in the past does not necessarily mean that it can't be tried again. Diseases change and may become more responsive to treatment.

What You Need to Ask Your Doctor

Do I really need this medication?

Some physicians decide to prescribe medications not because they are really necessary, but because they think patients want and expect drugs. Don't pressure your physician for medications. If your doctor doesn't prescribe a medication, consider that good news rather than a sign of rejection or indifference. Ask about nondrug alternatives. Many conditions can be treated in a variety of ways, and your physician can explain your options. In some cases, lifestyle changes such as exercise, diet, and stress management should be considered before other choices. When any treatment is recommended, ask what the likely consequences are if you postpone treatment. Sometimes the best medicine is none at all.

What is the name of the medication?

If a medication is prescribed, it is important that you know its name. Write down both the brand name and the generic (chemical) name. If the medication you get from the pharmacy doesn't have the same name as the one your doctor prescribed, ask the pharmacist to explain the difference.

What is the medication supposed to do?

Your doctor should tell you why the medication is being prescribed and how it might be expected to help you. Is the medication intended to prolong your life, completely or partially relieve your symptoms, or improve your ability to function? For example, if you are given an anti-HIV drug such as AZT (Retrovir), the purpose is primarily to prevent or slow deterioration of your immune system. It probably won't stop your HIV-related symptoms, and it may give you side effects. On the other hand, if you are given a skin cream, the purpose is to help ease your skin condition.

You should also know how soon you should expect results from the medication. Drugs that treat infections or inflammation may take several days to a week to show improvement, while antidepressant medications typically take several weeks to begin working.

How and when do I take the medication, and for how long?

Understanding how much of the medication to take and how often to take it is critical. Does "every 6 hours" mean "every 6 hours while awake"? Should the medication be taken before meals, with meals, or between meals? What should you do if you accidentally miss a dose? Should you skip it, take a double dose next time, or take it as soon as you remember? Should you continue taking the medication until the symptoms go away or until the medication is used up?

The answers to such questions are very important. For example, if you are taking an antibiotic for a lung infection, you may feel better within a few days, but you should continue taking the medication as prescribed to completely eliminate the infection; otherwise, the infection may come back, perhaps in a stronger, drug-resistant form. Didanosine (ddI, Videx) must be taken two pills at a time and chewed or crushed in order to be effective. If you are using an inhaled medication for breathing problems, the way you use the inhaler determines how much of the medication actually gets into your lungs. Taking medication properly is vital. Yet when patients are surveyed, nearly 40 percent report that they were not told by their physicians how to take the medication or how much to take. If you are not sure about your prescription, call your doctor. Such calls are never considered a bother.

What foods, drinks, other medications, or activities should I avoid while taking this medication?

Having food in your stomach may help protect the stomach from some medications, whereas it may render other drugs ineffective. For example, milk products or antacids can decrease the absorption of some drugs (such as Nizoral) but may increase the absorption of others (such as Fortovase). Some medications may make you more sensitive to the sun, putting you at increased risk for sunburn. Ask whether the medication prescribed will interfere with driving. Other drugs you may be taking, even OTC drugs and alcohol, can either amplify or lessen the effects of the prescribed medication. The more medications you are taking, the greater the chances of undesirable drug interactions. So ask about possible drug-drug and drug-food interactions.

What are the most common side effects, and what should I do if they occur?

All medications have side effects. You need to know what symptoms to be on the lookout for and what action to take if they develop. Should you seek immediate medical care, discontinue the medication, or call your doctor?

Although your doctor cannot be expected to list every possible adverse reaction, the more common and important ones should be discussed. Unfortunately, a recent survey showed that 70 percent of patients starting a new medication did not recall being told by their physicians or pharmacists about precautions and possible side effects. So it may be up to you to ask.

Are tests necessary to monitor the use of this medication?

Some medications are monitored by the improvement or worsening of symptoms. However, many medications used to treat people with HIV can disrupt body chemistry before any telltale symptoms develop. Sometimes these adverse reactions can be detected by laboratory tests such as blood counts or liver function tests. In addition, the levels of some medications in the blood need to be measured periodically to make sure you are getting the right amounts. Ask your doctor if the medication being prescribed has any of these special requirements.

Can a generic medication that is less expensive be prescribed?

Every drug has at least two names, a generic name and a brand name. The generic name is the nonproprietary, or chemical, name of the drug. The brand name is the manufacturer's unique name for the drug. When a drug company develops a new drug in the United States, it is granted exclusive rights to produce that drug for seventeen years. After the seventeen-year period has expired, other companies may market chemical equivalents of that drug. These generic medications are generally considered as safe and effective as the original brand-name drug but often cost half as much. Because many AIDS drugs are quite new, often no generic equivalent is available. Right now, there are no generic anti-HIV cocktail medications. Even so, if cost is a concern, ask your doctor if there is a lower-cost but equally effective medication. Sometimes you can save money by purchasing your medications through the mail. Many health maintenance organizations (HMOs) and mail-order pharmacies offer prescription services.

Is there any written information about the medication?

Realistically, your doctor may not have time to answer all of your questions in detail. Even if your physician carefully answers the questions, it is difficult for anyone to remember all this information. Fortunately, there are many other valuable sources of information you can turn to: pharmacists, nurses, package inserts, pamphlets, and books. Some particularly useful publications to consult are listed in the "Suggested Reading" section at the end of this chapter.

A Special Word about Pharmacists

Your pharmacist is an expert on medications. You can often call him or her on the phone to find out about medications and how they work. In addition, many hospitals, medical schools, and schools of pharmacy have medication information services you can call to ask questions. As a self-manager, don't forget pharmacists. They are important and helpful consultants.

Suggested Reading

Beach, Wayne A. *Conversation about Illness.* Hillsdale, N.J.: Lawrence Erlbaum Associates, 1996.

Jones, J. Alfred, Kreps, Gary L., and Phillips, Gerald M. *Communicating with Your Doctor: Getting the Most out of Health Care.* Creskill, N.J.: Hampton Press, 1995.

5 Making Treatment Decisions

HIV treatment has changed dramatically during the last few years. There are now more medications available to help people with HIV. While this is good, it has also made the decisions about when to start treatment and what medications to take more difficult.

One of the most important things that a person with HIV needs to be able to discuss with his or her doctor is when to start taking anti-HIV medications. The decision to start taking anti-HIV drugs is not simple. It's especially difficult for a person who feels well, with no symptoms from HIV. On the other hand, we know that high levels of virus in the blood make most people sick eventually, so it makes sense to want to lower the viral load.

The HIV medications now available are very good. They perform miracles for some people. But at the same time, taking medications is work. It requires effort to remember to take the pills, to follow all the instructions for taking them properly, to deal with any side effects or inconveniences that the medications cause, and generally to fit the medications into your daily routine. So in a way, the short answer to the question of when to start taking anti-HIV drugs is this: start on the drugs when you *want* to do it, and when you *can* do it. Of course, figuring these issues out isn't easy, and that's what each person with HIV has to work out with his or her doctor.

As you think about your decision, you and your doctor will want to consider both medical issues, related to the immune system and the virus, and personal issues, related to your own strengths and priorities. Later in this chapter we will look at some of the experts' recommendations for when people should think about using anti-HIV drugs and other treatments. But general recommendations don't always fit every individual. Here are some of the questions you'll need to talk through with your doctor:

- How much is your immune system already affected? What is the CD4+ or T cell count?

- How much risk is there of disease progression? What is the viral load (plasma HIV RNA level) now?
- How motivated are you to start the medications?
- After you've gotten all the help that's possible from your health care team, friends, and family, how likely is it—how confident are you—that you can take the anti-HIV medications exactly as they're supposed to be taken?
- Are the potential benefits of starting the medications greater than the risks?

Working out the answers to these questions may not be easy or straightforward. You may want to get the opinion of a second doctor, or talk with people who are already using the medications. But thinking about these issues and discussing them is really necessary so that you can make an informed decision.

Starting Anti-HIV Therapy

As we've said already, the time to start anti-HIV treatment is when you've thought about treatment, discussed it with your doctor, and *feel ready* to start. To decide when to start, it will help to consider the recommendations compiled by experts. The following table is based on recommendations from the Panel on Clinical Practices for Treatment of HIV Infection, convened by the U.S. Department of Health and Human Services and the Henry J. Kaiser Family Foundation. If you have HIV and you've never been on anti-HIV medications, take a look at the table, and bring it in to discuss with your doctor. It can be a good starting point for weighing the risks and benefits of treatment.

Other Treatments to Keep You Healthy

Even though the anti-HIV cocktail medications are important, they're certainly not the *only* important part of medical care for a person with HIV. A lot of the trouble people have with HIV is caused by opportunistic infections and cancers rather than by HIV itself. In theory, if we could prevent these oppor-

Making the Treatment Decision

Symptoms	T Cell Count and HIV Viral Load	Recommendation
AIDS, oral thrush, or fevers that are unexplained and don't go away	Any value	Treatment is recommended.
No symptoms	T cell count less than 500/microliter **or** HIVviral load greater than 10,000 (bDNA) or greater than 20,000 (RT-PCR)*	Treatment should be considered, with the decision based on whether the benefits of treatment are worth effort and risk.**
No symptoms	T cell count greater than 500/microliter **and** HIV viral load less than 10,000 (bDNA) or less than 20,000 (RT-PCR)*	Many experts recommend simply watching and waiting. Some, however, recommend that you consider treatment.

* bDNA is the branched-chain DNA test for viral load. RT-PCR is the reverse-transcriptase polymerase chain reaction test for viral load. Test results using bDNA run a bit lower than tests using RT-PCR, but either test is good if you read and interpret the results properly.

** Some experts would hold off on treatment for patients with T cell counts between 350 and 500 per microliter and HIV RNA levels less than 10,000 (bDNA) or less than 20,000 (RT-PCR).

tunistic infections and cancers from happening, people with HIV/AIDS could do quite well.

In addition to your cocktail medications, other strategies will help you prevent disease:

- Strengthen the immune system against infections with immunizations.
- Eliminate traces of infection with preventive antibiotics before the infection develops into disease.

- Detect signs of infection early, so that it can be treated before it causes problems.
- Adopt lifestyle changes that promote or maintain general good health.

To make sure you're getting the best care possible, you must stay up to date on your basic prevention strategies. The tables on the next few pages list the basic tests, medications, and vaccines that are recommended for adults with HIV/AIDS (children are different—don't use these guidelines for them). Remember, these are basic guidelines. For most people, these guidelines act as a minimum standard; many doctors and people with HIV/AIDS will do more than what is listed here. You and your doctor might decide to do things differently, depending on your circumstances. But if you decide *not* to do one of the things listed, it should be because you've thought about it, talked to your doctor about it, and made an informed and careful decision. That's the essence of being a self-manager.

To use the tables, look under the correct heading for your T cell count* and make sure that you and your doctor do each of the things listed. Prepare by making a list to bring to the doctor's office.

---

* We discuss T cells and the meaning of the various T cell counts in Chapter 3.

When You Begin Care for HIV (Any T Cell Count) . . .

Tests	Plasma HIV RNA concentration (HIV viral load)
	CD4+ T cell count (absolute T helper count and percent T helper count)
	Complete blood count (white blood cells, red blood cells, anemia, platelets)
	Complete blood chemistry profile
	Baseline syphilis blood test
	Baseline hepatitis B and C blood tests
	Toxoplasmosis antibody test
	Baseline chest x-ray
	Baseline vaginal and pelvic exam, and Pap test (women)
	Baseline oral/dental exam
	Baseline physical exam
	Skin test for tuberculosis (PPD* tuberculin test) and skin test for anergy**
Vaccines	Diptheria-tetanus (every 10 years)
	Pneumococcal vaccine (every 10 years)
	Influenza vaccine (every fall/winter)
	Hepatitis B vaccine if the hepatitis B blood test is negative (series of three shots once)
Medications	Evaluate your symptoms, viral load, and T cell count, and *discuss anti-HIV medications with your doctor* (see "Starting Anti-HIV Therapy," p. 54).
	If your PPD test is positive and there is no active TB, take isoniazid (INH) therapy for one year to prevent TB.
Self-care	Find a health care provider who you like and can talk to, and who knows about HIV. Think hard about changing your health habits—sex, smoking, alcohol, drugs.

*Purified protein derivative

**Anergy skin testing checks to make sure your immune system can respond to skin tests.

If Your T Cell Count Is Greater than 200 . . .

Tests	Plasma HIV RNA concentration (HIV viral load) every 3–6 months
	CD4+ T cell count every 3–6 months
	Syphilis blood test every year, or after new sexual exposure
	Prompt exam by eye doctor if vision problems develop
	Vaginal and pelvic exam, and Pap test (women) every 6–12 months
	Oral/dental exam every 6 months
	Routine physical exam every 6 months
	Skin tests for tuberculosis (PPD tuberculin test) and anergy every 6 months
Vaccines	Influenza vaccine (every fall/winter)
Medications	Evaluate your symptoms, viral load, and T cell count and *discuss anti-HIV medications with your doctor* (see "Starting Anti-HIV Therapy," p. 54).
	If your PPD test is positive and there is no active TB, take isoniazid (INH) therapy for one year to prevent TB.
Self-care	Educate yourself about HIV and the medications available.
	Build a partnership with your doctor.

If Your T Cell Count Is Less than 200 . . .

Tests

Plasma HIV RNA concentration (HIV viral load) every 3–6 months

CD4+ T cell count every 3–6 months

Syphilis blood test every year, or after new sexual exposure

Prompt exam by eye doctor if vision problems develop

Vaginal and pelvic exam, and Pap test (women) every 6–12 months

Oral/dental exam every 6 months

Routine physical exam every 6 months

Skin tests for tuberculosis (PPD tuberculin test) and anergy every 6 months

Vaccines

Influenza vaccine (every fall/winter)

Medications

Evaluate your symptoms, viral load, and T cell count and *discuss anti-HIV medications with your doctor* (see "Starting Anti-HIV Therapy," p. 54).

Take TMP/SMZ,* dapsone, or inhaled pentamidine to prevent *Pneumocystis* pneumonia.

If your PPD test is positive and there is no active TB, take isoniazid (INH) therapy for one year to prevent TB.

If your T cell count is less than 100 cells/µl, take TMP/SMZ* or dapsone-pyrimethamine to prevent toxoplasmosis.

If your T cell count is less than 50 cells/µl, take clarithromycin or azithromycin to prevent *Mycobacterium avium* complex (MAC).

Self-care

Educate yourself about HIV and the medications available.

Bulid a partnership with your doctor.

Make sure you know about your doctor's night/weekend coverage system, in case you need it.

Exercise and eat nutritious foods.

*Trimethoprim/sulfamethoxazole.

Suggested Reading

About Your Medicines. United States Pharmacopeial Convention, 1993.

AIDS Treatment News. ATN, P.O. Box 411256, San Francisco, CA 94141. (A semi-monthly newsletter reporting on HIV/AIDS treatments.) Published by John S. James.

The American Medical Association Guide to Prescription and Over-the-Counter Drugs. Chicago: American Medical Association, 1997.

Rybacki, James J., and Long, James W. *The Essential Guide to Prescription Drugs 2000* (serial). New York: Harper Resource, 1999.

Kearney, Brian, and Petrow, Steven (eds). *The HIV Drug Book.* New York: Pocket Books, 1998. (A comprehensive reference about many drugs used by people with HIV.)

6   Using Anti-HIV Medications

L ots of different types of medications are prescribed for people with HIV, including antibiotics that fight a variety of infections, and medications that treat symptoms such as pain and depression. But anti-HIV (antiretroviral) drugs are the ones that specifically attack HIV itself. These drugs are the main treatment for HIV, and improvement in these types of drugs in recent years has made a dramatic difference in many people's lives.

In this chapter we talk about how anti-HIV medications work and how they should be used. Of course, HIV treatment is complicated. Even experienced doctors and health care professionals need all their skills and knowledge to do it well. But a person with HIV needs to know the basics, too.

This chapter gives you the basics. There is a lot of other information about medications and treatment available—whole books have been devoted to the subject.* Our goal here is to give you a good starting point for talking with your doctor and doing more of your own research.

How Anti-HIV Medications Work

HIV lives in the body by making copies of itself, in a complicated series of chemical steps. If the virus *can't* copy itself, the immune system keeps it under control so that no HIV is detectable in the blood. As long as HIV isn't circulating in the blood, it can't damage the body further. Anti-HIV medications work by blocking the different steps that the virus uses to copy itself.

Reverse transcriptase is one of the chemicals HIV uses to copy itself, and many HIV drugs work by blocking reverse transcriptase. This is how *nucleoside* drugs,

---

* One such book is Project Inform's *The HIV Drug Book,* published by Pocket Books (1998).

such as zidovudine, lamivudine, and abacavir, work. The drugs "fool" the reverse transcriptase into trying to use them as raw material to make HIV copies, and by doing this they block the copying. Nonnucleoside reverse-transcriptase inhibitors (NNRTIs), such as Viramune and Sustiva, work by binding to reverse transcriptase and blocking its action.

Protease is a chemical that HIV uses fairly late in the process of copying itself. Drugs that block the protease *(protease inhibitors)* have proven to be very powerful anti-HIV agents and have become a crucial part of the cocktail combinations. Medications such as nelfinavir (Viracept), indinavir (Crixivan), and saquinavir (Fortovase) are all protease inhibitors.

If all these drugs block the copying of HIV, why is it important to use two, three, or four different drugs at the same time? The reason is that HIV has the ability to become resistant to drugs. People who take certain HIV drugs alone can develop resistant HIV within months—or even weeks, in some cases. Once a person develops resistance to an HIV drug, that drug won't work against the person's HIV ever again. Because drug-resistant HIV strains can be passed on to other people, drug resistance is a serious problem not only for that person, but for the larger population as well. But HIV cannot develop resistance to several drugs *when they're all used at the same time.* This is why multidrug treatment is important, and why having only one drug alone in your system is bad.

New blood tests are now coming into use that can detect and measure drug-resistant HIV in the blood. These tests, called HIV genotype and HIV phenotype tests, are still being studied and improved, but they may soon prove to be useful in HIV care. They could allow doctors to test a person who has used HIV drugs in the past to find out if he or she has become resistant to the drugs.

Adherence

"Adherence" means that after you and your doctor have agreed on what medications to try, *you stick to the medications exactly as they are prescribed by the doctor.* If it is impossible to stick to the medications because of side effects or for some other reason, you need to talk about the problem with the doctor right away. It's very important not to miss any pills, either by forgetting, intentionally skipping, or changing the schedule.

Adhering to HIV medications can be difficult for all sorts of reasons. For one thing, HIV treatment plans are usually very complicated. In research with people who have diseases that are much simpler than HIV (high blood pressure, for example), many people have difficulty adhering to even the simplest treatment plans. But HIV treatment is *not* simple; it may involve taking twenty-five pills each day, or even more. And some HIV medications must be taken on an empty stomach, while others must be taken with meals. All this can be difficult, especially for people who are sick, weak, or experiencing severe HIV symptoms. To make it even more difficult, HIV patients usually need to continue their treatments for a long time, perhaps indefinitely.

Side effects also can make it hard to stick with HIV treatment. Medications may cause problems such as nausea, headaches, diarrhea, tiredness, or dizziness. While it's much harder to stay on a medication that is causing side effects, it's not impossible. Many side effects ease off with time or can be managed using simple techniques. Some of these techniques are discussed later in this chapter.

For many people, the major problem with taking the medicines is that they just don't fit well into most daily routines. The medications aren't convenient, so doses are forgotten. You may sleep through a dose, you might be away from home, or be too busy, or simply forget.

Whether you're about to start HIV medications or you're already on cocktail drugs, there are things you can do to make your treatment successful.

If you are considering starting anti-HIV drugs . . .

1. *Play an active role in the treatment plan.* Ask your doctor to describe all your options, including the potential benefits and risks of starting treatment now instead of later. Also ask your doctor to explain any side effects or other problems that could be associated with the medication. If you're going to make the effort necessary to take these medications correctly, you need to understand the goals of treatment and how to achieve them.

2. *Let your doctor know about personal issues that could make it hard for you to take the medications.* Be honest. Some things, such as use of drugs or alcohol, or problems with housing or with mental illness, are not easy to talk about at all, but they should be discussed. Studies have shown that adherence may be more difficult—but not impossible—for people dealing with these kinds of problems. Adherence also may be more difficult for people who have very complex regimens or who have had problems taking medications in the past.

   Sometimes you can't be sure what the problems are going to be. Many people do a "dry run," practicing the treatment using jelly beans or candy instead of real pills. This can help you anticipate what problems could arise.

3. *Ask for a written copy of the treatment plan.* It's helpful to have a list that shows each medication, when and how much to take each time, and if it must be taken with food or on an empty stomach. Many doctors can give you a list that has pictures of the pills, so you won't get them confused.

4. Most important, *talk to your doctor about how to make your treatment fit your lifestyle.* For example, you might discuss how you can link the taking of medicines to certain things that you do each day—waking up in the morning, brushing your teeth, taking a child to school, leaving work, or watching a certain TV show. People who arrange their medication schedule around their daily routines adhere to their treatment plans more successfully than those who don't.

5. *Make sure you can make a commitment to the treatment plan.* Talk to your doctor about all your concerns. You may need to talk things over two or three times before you feel comfortable about starting the anti-HIV drugs.

If you are already on the anti-HIV drugs and want to do better at taking them . . .

There are lots of strategies you can try, and it's vital that you find one that works for you. Here are some ideas:

1. *Try keeping your medications where you'll see them.* Some people find it helpful to keep their first morning dose next to the alarm clock or the coffee pot. Others keep backup medication supplies at work or in a briefcase.

2. *Use daily or weekly pill boxes to organize your medications.* Some people like to count and set out a week's worth of medications at a time, with one box or space for each part of the day. It often works well to count out pills at the same time each week, like every Sunday night at bedtime.

3. *Plan ahead for weekends, holidays, and changes in routine.* Many studies have shown that weekends are a big problem for adherence. Decide ahead of time how you will remember to take all of your doses. Make a plan for remembering your medications, and write it out.

4. *Use timers, alarm clocks, or pagers to remind you when to take your medication.* Take each medication at the same time every day.

5. *Keep a medication diary.* You can write the names of your drugs on a small card or in your daily planner, and then check off each dose as you take it.

6. *Get help and support from your family and friends.* You don't always have to go it alone. If you can, ask family members, friends, or loved ones to remind you to take your medication. Some people also find it helpful to join an HIV support group.

7. *Don't run out of medication.* Be sure to call your doctor or clinic if your supply will not last until your next visit.

Managing Side Effects

Medication side effects are a very big issue in HIV treatments. Patients and doctors have to figure out how to manage side effects and how to decide when they are dangerous, when they will improve on their own, and when they are so bothersome that the medications should be changed. Luckily, many side effects *can* be managed, so that you won't have to stop the medication and give up its benefits.

A special problem that many people experience is a change in the distribution of fat in the body. This is sometimes called "protease belly" or "buffalo hump," but the medical term is *lipodystrophy.* Both men and women may have wasting of the face, arms, and legs, along with deposits of fat around the middle of the body and at the base of the neck. Women's breasts may get very large due to fatty deposits, causing real problems with comfort and clothing. Although anyone with HIV can have lipodystrophy, it seems to be more common in people using protease inhibitor medications.

People who take protease inhibitors can also have increased levels of fat and cholesterol in the blood, and may have higher blood sugar. These problems cause some people a lot of embarrassment and discomfort. Sometimes it's necessary to use other medications to lower the levels of fat ("lipids") in the blood or to treat the high blood sugar. Chapter 11 provides some tips on how to cut back on fat and sugar in the diet. People who have abnormal concentrations of fat in the blood may want to use these tips to change their eating habits, and should find out from the doctor if other treatment is needed.

The table on page 66 lists some of the other side effects that have been associated with anti-HIV medications and gives some self-management techniques to try. Even if you have success in managing your side effects, though, remember to

Techniques for Managing Side Effects

Side Effect	What You Should Do
Diarrhea	This is a very common side effect, especially in the first few weeks of taking a new medication. It often goes away on its own.

- Eat plenty of fiber (vegetables) and drink lots of liquids (water).
- Eat more rice and other starches.
- Avoid dairy products (milk, ice cream, cheese).
- Consider switching to a low-fat diet.
- Ask your doctor about Metamucil, Lomotil, Imodium, or tincture of opium.
- **Keep your doctor or primary care provider informed.**

Fatigue

This is a very common side effect, especially in the first few weeks of taking a new medication. It often goes away on its own.

- Take frequent, short naps and try to sleep longer at night.
- Limit caffeine and sugar.
- Limit work hours, if possible. Try relaxation techniques.*
- Do light exercise (e.g., 15 to 30 minutes of brisk walking).
- **Keep your doctor or primary care provider informed.**

"Feeling different"

Many patients feel different, as if their thinking process or perception of the world has changed. Some will feel almost as if they're dreaming. This is a very common side effect, especially in the first few weeks of a regimen. It often goes away on its own.

- Try relaxation techniques.*
- Increase your sleep time and try short naps.
- Avoid alcohol and other drugs.
- Do light exercise (e.g., 15 to 30 minutes of brisk walking).
- **Keep your doctor or primary care provider informed.**

Headache

This is a very common side effect, especially in the first few weeks of taking a new medication. It often goes away on its own.

- Take Tylenol, aspirin, or Advil.
- Try relaxation techniques,* herbal teas, and soft music.
- **Keep your doctor or primary care provider informed.**

Nausea This is a very common side effect, especially in the first few weeks of taking a new medication. It often goes away on its own.

- Eat crackers, and sip ginger ale or other soft drinks.
- Eat cold or room-temperature foods and liquids.
- Try Mylanta or Maalox (not with medications).
- Avoid spicy foods and foods with lots of acid (e.g., oranges, tomatoes).
- Ask your doctor about Zofran, Compazine, and benzodiazepines.
- **Keep your doctor or primary care provider informed.**

If you are using ddI:

- Try crushing and dissolving pills in ice-cold water or juice.
- Try taking pills at a different time (like at bedtime).
- Remember that ddI must be taken on an empty stomach.

Numbness or tingling This is a very common side effect, which often goes away on its own.

- Eat a balanced diet and take a multivitamin each day.
- Tell your doctor or primary care provider if there is an increase in numbness or in the size of the numb area.

Rash This is a very common side effect, especially in the first few weeks of taking a new medication. It often goes away on its own, **but** it is very important that you see your doctor.

- **Talk to your doctor or primary care provider about "urgent" follow-up.**
- Report increasing rash, fever, headache, flu-like symptoms, or any sores in your mouth or vagina.
- Benadryl may help with itching (but use it **only** with your doctor's approval).

*Relaxation techniques are described in Chapter 9. Many bookstores have books or cassette tapes that can assist you.

keep your doctors and nurses informed about new symptoms, and especially any severe ones. You should also check the symptom action charts in Chapter 7, which can help you to determine whether a symptom is a side effect or whether it may be a sign of a serious illness.

Deciding When to Try a New Regimen

Just like deciding about when to start anti-HIV medications, deciding when to switch to a new combination of medicines is something that must be done very carefully, and always with the help of your doctor. Jumping from one set of medications to another too often can "use up" all your medication options, due to problems of resistance that we discussed earlier. But often, changing medications will be necessary, and this will be an important time for you to talk carefully with your doctor.

Although there are many factors to consider, in general there are two reasons why you might stop one set of anti-HIV medications and start another:

1. *Your current medications aren't working.* The job of the medications is to suppress the HIV in your blood, to boost or maintain your T cell count, and to keep you from getting HIV-related infections. If some of these things aren't being done well enough, it may be time to switch. This is pretty obvious, but what isn't obvious is where to draw the line—how low should the viral load number be for your medicines to be considered successful? If your numbers have been low, how much of an increase should cause you to decide to make a change? How much of a drop in the T cell count should make you change? The main point to keep in mind is that if the numbers are going in the "wrong" direction (up for viral load, down for T cells) and they're consistent on consecutive blood tests, then you and your doctor should talk about it. Depending on your situation, either staying on your medication or switching might be the right decision.

2. *Your current medications are too toxic.* It could be that your anti-HIV drugs are suppressing HIV very well and boosting your T cells, but that one or more of the drugs are making you so sick that you have to change. If you find this happening to you, talk with your doctor right away. Otherwise, you may wind up skipping or "forgetting" doses, and put yourself at risk for resis-

tance. And only you know what your side effects are like and if they're severe enough to warrant a change of medications. Although there are more treatment options now than ever before, the choices are still limited in many cases, so it's important to balance side effects against benefits when you make your decision.

Anti-HIV Medications: Standard Dosages and Common Side Effects

Following are tables that list the anti-HIV medications available now, along with the most common dosages and some of the side effects that may occur.*

---

*These tables and the drug information provided have been adapted from *Standard Dosing Schedule for Anti-HIV Drugs,* Project Inform, San Francisco, 1999.

Protease Inhibitors

Generic Name	Brand Name	Standard Dose*	Doses per Day	How to Take	Common Side Effects
Amprenavir	Agenerase	1200 mg (8 pills of 150 mg)	2	With or without food	Rash, fatigue, vomiting, headache, and diarrhea. Refer to pp. 65–68 for tips on managing these side effects.
Indinavir	Crixivan	800 mg (2 pills of 400 mg)	3	On an empty stomach, at least 1 hour before or 2 hours after a meal Every 8 hours Do not take at the same time as ddI. If combined with ddI, take 1 hour before or 2 hours after ddI.	Kidney stones. Drink at least 8 glasses of water daily to reduce this risk.

		Dose	Times daily	Food instructions	Side effects/notes
Nelfinavir	Viracept	750 mg (3 pills of 250 mg)	3	With food	Diarrhea and nausea. Refer to pp. 65–68 for tips on managing these side effects.
Ritonavir	Norvir	600 mg (6 pills of 100 mg)	2	Start gradually, first with 300 mg twice daily for 2 days, 400 mg twice daily for 2 days, 500 mg twice daily for 2 days, then on to the full dose of 600 mg twice daily.	Diarrhea and nausea, which are usually worse in the first few weeks of starting the medication. Refer to pp. 65–68 for tips on managing these side effects.
Saquinavir	Fortovase (soft gel)	1200 mg (6 pills of 200 mg)	3	With food, preferably within 2 hours of eating a high-fat meal	People with liver problems should be careful using this drug.
	Invirase (hard)	600 mg (3 pills of 200 mg)	3		Diarrhea and nausea. Refer to pp. 65–68 for tips on managing these side effects.

*It may be necessary to modify the dose of one or more drugs in a combination when taking a protease inhibitor or an NNRTI with another protease inhibitor or NNRTI and other common over-the-counter and prescription medications.

Nonnucleoside Reverse-Transcriptase Inhibitors (NNRTIs)

Generic Name	Brand Name	Standard Dose*	Doses per Day	How to Take	Common Side Effects
Efavirenz	Sustiva	600 mg (3 pills of 200 mg)	1	With or without food. Take at night to reduce chances of neurological side effects. Pregnant women should not take this drug.	Neurological symptoms, such as dizziness, drowsiness, and lack of concentration. Refer to pp. 65–68 for tips on managing these side effects.
Delavirdine	Rescriptor	400 mg (4 pills of 100 mg)	3	With or without food. Can be dissolved in water or other liquids if drank immediately.	Rash, which usually appears within first 3 weeks of treatment. Refer to pp. 65–68 for tips on managing this side effect. If the rash becomes severe, hospitalization may be needed.

| Nevirapine | Viramune | 200 mg (1 pill) | 2 | With or without food. Dose is increased over first 2 weeks, starting with 1 (200 mg) pill daily and then 2 pills daily after 14 days. | Rash, which usually appears within first 3 weeks of treatment. Refer to pp. 65–68 for tips on managing this side effect. If the rash becomes severe, hospitalization may be needed. |

*It may be necessary to modify the dose of one or more drugs in a combination when taking a protease inhibitor or an NNRTI with another protease inhibitor or NNRTI and other common over-the-counter and prescription medications.

Nucleoside Analogue Reverse-Transcriptase Inhibitors (NARTIs)

Generic Name	Brand Name	Standard Dose*	Doses Per Day	How to Take	Common Side Effects
Abacavir	Ziagen	300 mg (1 pill)	2	With or without food	Nausea, vomiting, headache, and fatigue. Refer to pp. 65–68 for tips on managing these side effects. About 3% of people develop a hypersensitivity to this drug, which causes flu-like symptoms. If this happens, contact the doctor immediately. The drug should be stopped and not taken again to avoid severe side effects.

Zidovudine	AZT, Retrovir	200 mg (2 pills of 100 mg) or 300 mg (1 pill)	3 2	With or without food	Headache, nausea, and sense of feeling ill. These usually subside after 6 to 8 weeks. Refer to pp. 65–68 for tips on managing these side effects. Anemia is the most serious side effect, which is treatable if caught early.
Zidovudine + lamivudine	Combivir	150 mg lamivudine (1 pill) and 300 mg zidovudine (1 pill)	2	With or without food	See side effects for both zidovudine and lamivudine.
Zalcitabine	ddC, Hivid	0.75 mg (1 pill)	3	With or without food	Pain or tingling in feet and/or hands (peripheral neuropathy), low blood platelets (thrombocytopenia) and mouth sores.

*It may be necessary to modify the dose of one or more drugs in a combination when taking a protease inhibitor or an NNRTI with another protease inhibitor or NNRTI and other common over-the-counter and prescription medications.

(continued)

Generic Name	Brand Name	Standard Dose*	Doses per Day	How to Take	Common Side Effects
Zalcitabine (*cont.*)					Pancreatitis is the most serious side effect. Symptoms include sharp pain in upper part of the abdomen, nausea, and vomiting. Stop drug immediately and call your doctor. Alcohol use increases risk of pancreatitis.
Didanosine	ddI, Videx	200 mg (2 pills of 100 mg)	2	On an empty stomach Cannot be taken within 2 hours of drugs that require acid in the stomach, such as many of the protease inhibitors.	Increased uric acid levels, headaches, sleeplessness, diarrhea, and pain or tingling in feet and/or hands. Refer to pp. 65–68 for tips on managing these.

					Pancreatitis can also be a serious side effect. See side effects from zalcitabine.
Stavudine	d4T, Zerit	40 mg (1 pill)	2	With or without food	Pain or tingling in the feet and/or hands, anemia. Rare incidence of pancreatitis. See side effects from zalcitabine.
Lamivudine	3TC, Epivir	150 mg (1 pill)	2	With or without food	Headaches, nausea, sense of feeling ill, diarrhea, anemia, and hair loss. Refer to pp. 65–68 for tips on managing some of these effects.

*It may be necessary to modify the dose of one or more drugs in a combination when taking a protease inhibitor or an NNRTI with another protease inhibitor or NNRTI and other common over-the-counter and prescription medications.

In addition to these anti-HIV medications there is another type, called a *nucleotide analogue reverse transcriptase inhibitor (NtARTI)*. Adefovir (Preveon) and tenofovir are two such drugs. Currently, they are available only through drug studies and early access programs.

Suggested Reading and Resources

Refer to the readings and resources listed for Chapters 3 and 5.

Managing Your Symptoms

7

Evaluating Common Symptoms of HIV/AIDS

Symptoms are the body's signals that something unusual is happening, that something is not right. They cannot always be seen by others, are often difficult to describe, and are usually unpredictable. Having HIV/AIDS means that you are probably going to have symptoms that will need to be managed. Although some symptoms are common, when and how they affect each of us is very personal. Also, symptoms such as fatigue, stress, shortness of breath, pain, anger, depression, and sleep disturbances can interact with each other, which in turn worsens health and leads to the development of new symptoms.

Although the chronic symptoms of HIV/AIDS are difficult to live with, there are many things you can learn to help you deal with them better. In this chapter we will look at how to evaluate some of the common symptoms associated with HIV/AIDS so that you can decide whether a symptom needs immediate medical attention. If you have not experienced any symptoms, this information will help prepare you for what to expect if symptoms do begin. It will also help you determine if symptoms are part of a normal illness, such as a common cold or the flu, or if they are something more serious. In Chapter 8, we will discuss the more common chronic symptoms of HIV/AIDS and some of their causes, and in Chapter 9 we will present some specific suggestions for dealing with these symptoms, particularly those techniques that involve the use of the mind.

In general, people with HIV/AIDS can view their symptoms as falling in three broad groups.

First, some symptoms are medication *side effects*—symptoms caused by the medications themselves. Side effects are variable. A side effect that is quite severe in one person may be very mild for someone else. And, of course, different medications have different side effects. Side effects are particularly common with "cocktail" anti-HIV medications. It may seem as if dealing with side effects is a simple matter—stop the medications that cause the side effects, and switch to something else. But for most people, there are no perfect drug combinations with no side effects at all. So to get the benefit of the medications, it's important to *balance* the side effects against the good things the medicines do, and manage them as well as possible. We've already discussed some side effect symptoms and management strategies in Chapter 4.

Second, new symptoms could be caused by *a new HIV-related infection*. For example, a new cough with fever could be a symptom of pneumonia. People who have symptoms that might be from new infections need to see the doctor right away, because detecting these conditions and starting treatment early is vital. The symptom action charts included later in this chapter are designed to help people decide when it's important to see the doctor.

Third, many *chronic conditions* (including chronic HIV) obviously can cause symptoms themselves. People with arthritis may get joint or back pains, people with chronic lung disease may become short of breath, and people with HIV may develop fatigue or other symptoms. People with chronic disease experience chronic symptoms that may increase and decrease but that can be managed with a good program for living well.

In addition to helping you deal with your disease symptoms, the various techniques described throughout the book will also help you to live well by maintaining health and slowing or preventing the onset of new symptoms.

Keep the following suggestions in mind when trying out a self-management technique and planning your self-management program:

- *Read all three chapters on symptoms and their management* (Chapters 7–9).

- *Evaluate each new symptom.* Symptoms are always distressing, but sometimes they are important clues that something new is happening that needs to be addressed. A new or worsening symptom could be a sign of a drug side effect or an opportunistic infection.* To be an effective self-manager, you need to know when it's okay to use home self-management techniques and when you should see the doctor.

- *Pick one technique to try first.* Be sure to give it a fair trial. We recommend that you practice the technique for at least two weeks, twice a day, before deciding whether it is going to be helpful to you. Also try some of the other techniques, giving each the same trial period. It is important to try more than one technique, because some may be more useful for a particular symptom, or you may find that you simply prefer some techniques over others.

---

*"Opportunistic infection" is a general term for all of the serious infections associated with HIV.

- *After choosing the techniques you like, think about how and when you will use each one.* This will depend on exactly what you're trying to accomplish. Some techniques are specific to certain symptoms; for example, certain diet changes may be appropriate for managing diarrhea, whereas inhaling moist heat is good for nasal congestion. Some of the exercises can be done anywhere, whereas others require a quiet place. Some may require substantial lifestyle changes. Also, you may find in your practice of the different techniques that some work well for certain symptoms but not so well for other symptoms. The best symptom managers learn to use a variety of techniques tailored to their needs and situations.

- *Finally, because practice and consistency are important for the mastery of some of these techniques, place cues in your environment to remind you to practice them.* For example, place a sticker or note where you'll see it, such as on your mirror, in your office, next to your medicines, on the car's dashboard, or near your home phone. You can change the stickers or notes periodically so you will continue to notice them. Also, try linking these new activities to some other established behavior or activity in your daily routine. For example, practice relaxation as part of your cooldown from exercise. You might ask a friend, family member, or partner to remind you to get your practice in each day; they may even wish to participate.

Evaluating Your Symptoms

One of the distressing things about living with HIV is that one is always concerned about developing an AIDS-related infection or other condition. New symptoms, especially if they are your first symptoms, are distressing in and of themselves, and also because they could be signals of a new or more serious problem. The truth is that symptoms sometimes *can* be signals that a serious illness is starting and you should see your doctor. Just as often, however, the symptoms are part of the vicious cycle of chronic disease, for which self-management may be the best approach.

To feel confident in using self-management, you need to know when it's time to call the doctor. But how can you tell? Some of it is common sense. If it's clear you're having a medical emergency, see a doctor immediately. On the other hand, if you're having symptoms similar to what you've often had in the past, you can probably use self-management techniques confidently.

Side effects can be tricky to evaluate, because sometimes a new symptom will start after you begin a medication, but it isn't caused by the medication. In rare cases, you could be on a medication for months or even years before a side effect occurs. But usually you can tell you're having a side effect if new symptoms begin after you start a new medication and go away after you stop the medication.

Another important factor in evaluating symptoms is to know your T cell count (also called CD4+ cell count). T cells are one way of estimating the strength of the immune system; people with a T-cell count lower than 200 are usually at higher risk for getting infections, so they have to be more careful. Your doctor should measure your T cell count at least every six months, and it's a good idea to know the result of your most recent measurement. Of course, T cells aren't the only measure of how healthy you are, but they are useful. There's more information about T cells in Chapter 3.

One quick way to judge whether you should see your doctor for a symptom is to do a FAST check. Ask yourself the four simple questions listed in the following chart. If the answer to any of the questions is yes, you should see your doctor promptly. He or she will be able to tell you if the symptom is due to a new AIDS-related infection or cancer.

Fever

Fever can be a chronic symptom in HIV/AIDS, but it also can be an important clue when it appears in association with another symptom. A temperature of 101°F (38.3°C) is more likely to be associated with infection.

Do a FAST Check on All New or Worsening Symptoms	
Fever	Is the new symptom associated with a fever (a temperature of 101°F or more)?
Altered mental status	Is the new symptom associated with alteration in mental status (confusion, sleepiness, seizures)?
Severe	Is the new symptom much more severe than anything you've had in the past?
Typical	Is the new symptom *not* typical for you?

Note: *Everyone* with HIV needs to own, and know how to use, a thermometer. It is important to *measure* your temperature when you think you have a fever. *Write down* the temperature so you will be able to tell the doctor if necessary.

Altered Mental Status

The brain is the body's most important organ, so it is a sensitive indicator of when trouble is present. *Altered mental status* is a term doctors use to describe a person whose brain functioning is not normal. This can mean confusion, excessive sleepiness, or "I can't put my finger on it, but he just isn't himself." It can also take a much more dramatic form, such as a coma (the most extreme decrease in mental function) or a seizure. All of these conditions represent altered mental status. Anyone who develops new altered mental status, particularly in association with other symptoms, should see a doctor promptly.

You may not be able to recognize a serious alteration in mental function yourself, but you can teach those close to you how to easily diagnose such a change. If they suspect you may be subject to an altered mental status, they should simply see how well you answer questions. If you can't answer questions coherently or can't wake up enough to answer them, urgent action is needed.

Severe

Chronic symptoms will often increase and decrease depending on whether you're having a good day or a bad day. However, any symptom that is much more severe than it has ever been before should be evaluated by your health care team.

Typical

Any symptom that is completely new for you (that is *not typical*) should be discussed with your medical team. This is a very general guideline that you probably use already when deciding whether to go to the doctor. Depending on what the new symptom is, you may want to consult one of the symptom action charts that follow for more guidance. But remember that when in doubt, it's better to be safe than sorry. If you're experiencing a symptom you've never had before and you're not sure whether self-care is the right thing to do, it's best to consult your doctor to be sure.

Using Symptom Action Charts

Another way to evaluate your symptoms is to use action charts. These charts will guide you in evaluating several common HIV/AIDS-related symptoms that sometimes require a doctor's rapid attention. Not every symptom is included here, but if you have one of the symptoms listed, the chart will help you decide what to do.

If you have more than one symptom, you may need to look at more than one chart. If the advice doesn't agree between the two charts, follow the most "conservative" (that is, the safest) advice. For example, if one chart says to call the doctor and the other recommends home treatment, you should call your doctor.

If you use the charts properly by following the steps below, they will guide you through the key questions you should consider in deciding whether you need the help of your health care team right away.

1. *Determine your "chief complaint"* or symptom, and then find the correct chart. (They are arranged alphabetically.)
2. Before you look at the chart, *read the general information* on the symptom opposite the chart. This information will help you understand the questions in the chart. If you ignore the general information, you may not understand the questions in the chart correctly, and you could do the wrong thing.
3. *Read the action chart.* Start at the top and follow the arrows. Skipping around may result in errors. Each question assumes that you have answered all of the previous questions.

    Note: These charts are intended only to help you decide if you need to see your doctor urgently for certain symptoms. Regardless of symptoms, you should always go in for the routine check-ups that you and your doctor have scheduled.

Cough

The *cough reflex* is a defense mechanism used by the body to clear abnormal material from the lungs. When the cough is bringing up infected material, such as pus, from the lungs, coughing is beneficial and shouldn't be suppressed. However, anything that irritates the lungs will cause a cough, and many of these stimuli do not produce pus, or even anything that's particularly easy to get out. So the cough will continue but not produce anything, and it can be quite aggravating.

Cough *can* be a medication side effect, but the medications most commonly associated with this are for blood pressure or heart disease (captopril, fosinopril, lisinopril, enalapril). For most people with HIV, a new cough is related to something else.

People with HIV/AIDS get coughs for all the same reasons other people do. Smoking is probably the most common cause; the toxins in the smoke irritate and kill cells in the linings of the bronchial tubes (breathing tubes) and stimulate the cough. This can happen even to those who don't smoke themselves but who breathe other people's smoke. Viral infections ("colds") are the next most

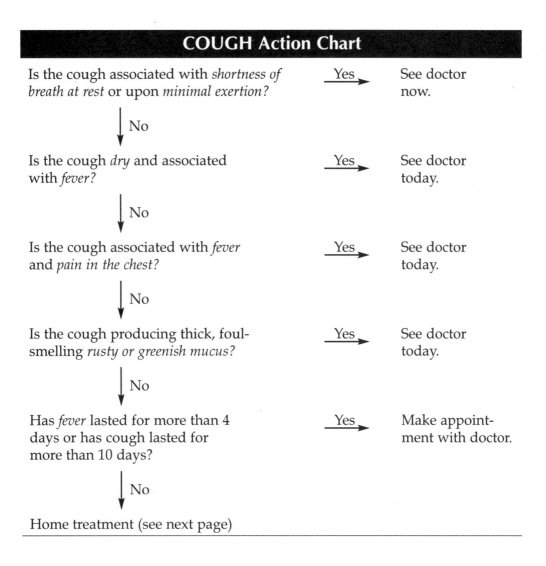

COUGH Action Chart

Is the cough associated with *shortness of breath at rest* or upon *minimal exertion?* — **Yes** → See doctor now.

↓ No

Is the cough *dry* and associated with *fever?* — **Yes** → See doctor today.

↓ No

Is the cough associated with *fever* and *pain in the chest?* — **Yes** → See doctor today.

↓ No

Is the cough producing thick, foul-smelling *rusty or greenish mucus?* — **Yes** → See doctor today.

↓ No

Has *fever* lasted for more than 4 days or has cough lasted for more than 10 days? — **Yes** → Make appointment with doctor.

↓ No

Home treatment (see next page)

common cause. These coughs usually produce only yellow or whitish mucus, not the green or rusty stuff produced by a more serious bacterial infection. Cold viruses don't respond to antibiotics; the only treatment is to strengthen the body's immune response with rest, good food, and lots of fluids. Bacterial infections can be more serious and require a doctor's attention and antibiotics.

In addition to the usual causes of cough, people with HIV/AIDS are susceptible to lung diseases not usually seen in people with stronger immune systems. The most common and most important of these is *Pneumocystis carinii* pneumonia (PCP). Identifying this disease early is vital because it is very dangerous when advanced. When caught early, however, it responds very well to antibiotics. The signs of PCP are a *dry cough* with *shortness of breath* and *fever*. Other lung infections that are seen in people with HIV/AIDS include tuberculosis (TB) and bacterial pneumonia. TB is a very serious lung disease that may cause a chronic cough with fevers yet may not cause much trouble with breathing. Unfortunately, TB is very easy to pass on to other people by coughing. Because of the risk of TB, you should bring any persistent cough (lasting longer than ten days) to the attention of your doctor.

Infection in the sinuses (*sinusitis*) doesn't affect the lungs directly, but it often causes coughing because mucus from the sinuses drips down the throat into the lungs, irritating them. This is particularly a problem at night.

Home Treatment of Cough

The mucus in the bronchial tubes may be made thinner and less sticky by several means. Increasing the humidity in the air will help; a vaporizer and a steamy shower are two ways to add humidity. Drinking a lot of fluids is helpful, particularly if a fever has dehydrated the body. Glyceryl guaiacolate (Robitussin) may help liquefy mucus so it can be coughed out of the lungs more easily. Decongestants (Sudafed) and/or antihistamines (Benadryl) may help if the cough is caused by nasal or sinus material dripping down into the lungs. (**Note:** These medicines should otherwise be avoided because they dry the mucus and make it thicker.*)

Dry, tickling coughs are often relieved by sucking on cough lozenges or hard candy. Dextromethorphan (Robitussin-DM) is an effective cough suppressant that you can buy without a prescription, but neither this nor codeine (available only with a prescription) will completely get rid of a cough, even at a high dosage.

---

*Over-the-counter cold medicines almost always contain antihistamine—and/or decongestant and/or expectorant—in some bewildering combination.

Diarrhea

Many of the concerns with diarrhea are the same as those with nausea and vomiting (see page 94). *Dehydration* is the greatest risk and can require intravenous medicines when it gets severe. Diarrhea that is *jet black* or *bloody* may indicate bleeding from the intestines. Most people with diarrhea will have cramping and intermittent gas-like pains, but *severe, steady abdominal pain* could be more serious.

In people with HIV/AIDS, diarrhea can be caused by viral, bacterial, or parasitic infections and is often caused by the effect of HIV itself on the intestines. In many cases, it is a side effect of a drug. Several anti-HIV medicines can cause diarrhea, including nelfinavir (Viracept), ritonavir (Norvir), amprenavir (Agenerase), and didanosine (ddI, Videx). Antibiotics and anticancer drugs also

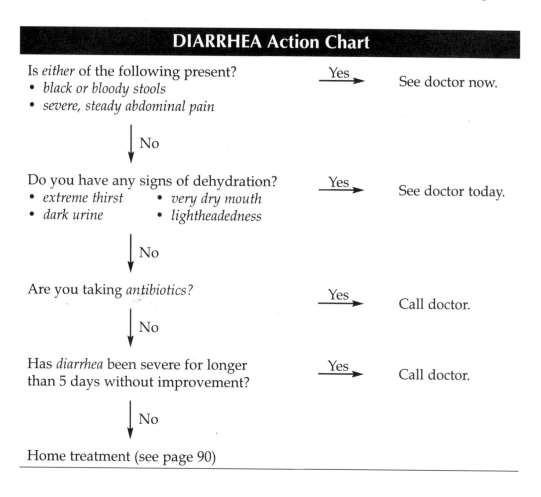

DIARRHEA Action Chart

Is *either* of the following present? — Yes → See doctor now.
- *black or bloody stools*
- *severe, steady abdominal pain*

No

Do you have any signs of dehydration? — Yes → See doctor today.
- *extreme thirst*   • *very dry mouth*
- *dark urine*   • *lightheadedness*

No

Are you taking *antibiotics?* — Yes → Call doctor.

No

Has *diarrhea* been severe for longer than 5 days without improvement? — Yes → Call doctor.

No

Home treatment (see page 90)

cause diarrhea in some people. If medications seem to be responsible for diarrhea, it is important to discuss this with the doctor.

Home Treatment of Diarrhea

Home treatment of diarrhea is directed at getting enough fluid into the body to prevent dehydration. Sip clear fluids, such as water or ginger ale. If you are vomiting and nothing else will stay down, suck on ice chips; this is usually tolerated and provides some fluids. Gatorade, bouillon, and Jell-O are also good sources of liquid. The next step is to move on to constipating foods: the "BRAT" rule of *bananas, rice, applesauce,* and *toast.* Milk and fats will not absorb well and should be avoided for a few days. Nonprescription remedies such as Kaopectate will make the stool more solid, but they won't change the amount or frequency of the stools. Many cases of diarrhea will get better on their own within five days, but if this doesn't happen, you should call your doctor. You may eventually need stronger medication to slow down the intestinal tract.

Fever

The most common cause of fevers in HIV/AIDS is infection. Probably the single most common cause of fever is HIV itself. Fever can be due to viral, bacterial, and parasitic infections and sometimes is due to cancers or medications. Fever is a distressing symptom, but it's rarely dangerous in itself. However, the infection that might be causing the fever could be very serious. Everyone needs to know how to measure a fever and how to decide when it's time to see the doctor.

If you have HIV, you should have a thermometer and know how to use it properly. Both Fahrenheit and centigrade thermometers are okay. If your temperature is greater than or equal to 101°F, it's important to consider whether you could have one of the serious, emergency AIDS-associated infections. These include meningitis, an infection of the lining of the brain that causes *neck stiffness* and *confusion,* and *Pneumocystis* pneumonia, an infection of the lungs that causes *dry cough* and *shortness of breath,* particularly upon exertion. People with a permanent central intravenous line (usually inserted into the upper arm or the chest) are at risk for bacterial sepsis (blood poisoning) and should be evaluated promptly upon developing *new fevers.*

If none of these problems is present, the fever still could be serious but probably doesn't require immediate attention by a doctor. The important consideration is what symptoms are associated with the fever and how they should be managed.

FEVER Action Chart

Is your temperature greater than or equal to 101°F (38.3°C) and associated with
- *neck stiffness?*
- *lethargy or confusion?*
- *seizure?*
- *severe irritability?*

Yes → See doctor now.

↓ No

Is your temperature greater than or equal to 101°F (38.3°C) and associated with *dry cough and severe shortness of breath?*

Yes → See doctor now.

↓ No

Is this a *new fever,* and are you using a central IV (intravenous) line for medications?

Yes → Call or see doctor today.

↓ No

Is the *fever* associated with a new *skin rash* or *skin sores?*

Yes → Call or see doctor today.

↓ No

Is the *fever* associated with
- *headache?*
- *cough* (not short of breath)?
- *sore throat?*
- *diarrhea?*
- *urinary problems?*

Yes → See section on the associated problem.

↓ No

Home treatment (see page 92)

Home Treatment of Fever

There are two ways to reduce a fever: sponging and medication. Sponging the skin with tepid water will bring the body temperature down as the water evaporates. Medications to lower fever include aspirin, acetaminophen (Tylenol, Datril), and ibuprofen (Motrin, Advil). Adults can take two aspirins every three to four hours as required. Acetaminophen is taken similarly and is often confused with aspirin, but it is a completely different medicine. It has the same effect as aspirin by lowering the temperature but causes less stomach upset. On the other hand, acetaminophen can cause liver damage in high doses, and overdose can be fatal. Since aspirin and acetaminophen are different drugs, they can be given together to control fever when one or the other alone is not effective. To do this, stagger the doses every three hours, alternating doses of aspirin and acetaminophen.

Headache

Headache is the single most frequent complaint of modern times. The most common causes of headache are tension (something that people with HIV/AIDS often have) and muscle spasms. Medications can also lead to headaches; zidovudine (AZT) is a frequent cause for some people.

However, there are several opportunistic diseases that can start out as headaches in people with HIV/AIDS. Headache associated with *fever* and a *neck so stiff that the chin cannot be touched to the chest* suggests the possibility of meningitis, a serious infection of the lining of the brain. Headaches could be caused by infection or a tumor in the brain itself if they are associated with neurological problems such as *slurred speech, weakness or paralysis in the arms or the legs,* or new *visual problems*. And any headache that comes after a *severe head injury* could be serious.

Home Treatment of Headache

The usual over-the-counter drugs (aspirin, acetaminophen, ibuprofen) are quite effective in relieving headache. Headache also responds very well to techniques that help reduce stress and tension. Try massage or heat applied to the back of the upper neck, or simply rest with your eyes closed and your head supported. Meditation is often effective. Headaches that don't respond to these measures should be brought to the attention of a doctor.

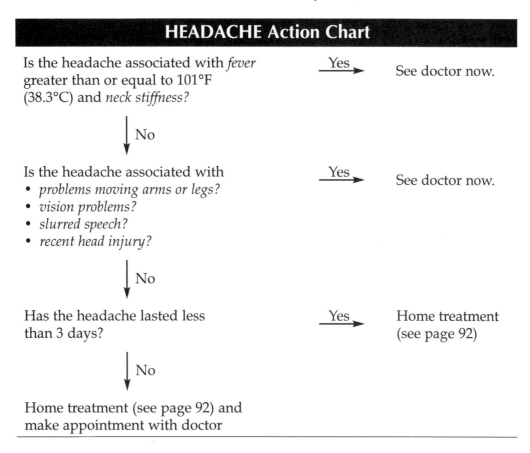

HEADACHE Action Chart

Is the headache associated with *fever* greater than or equal to 101°F (38.3°C) and *neck stiffness?*   ——Yes——▸   See doctor now.

↓ No

Is the headache associated with
- *problems moving arms or legs?*
- *vision problems?*
- *slurred speech?*
- *recent head injury?*

——Yes——▸   See doctor now.

↓ No

Has the headache lasted less than 3 days?   ——Yes——▸   Home treatment (see page 92)

↓ No

Home treatment (see page 92) and make appointment with doctor

Impaired/Decreased Vision

Your vision is important, so any vision change should lead you to see the doctor if it doesn't improve on its own. The most common causes of vision problems in people with HIV/AIDS are no different than in other people: nearsightedness and farsightedness. Also, sometimes vision will be affected by medications, headaches, eye strain, or fatigue. When one of these things is causing vision problems, the change is usually gradual and about equal in both eyes. You should see a doctor, but it isn't an emergency. But HIV/AIDS also can lead to CMV (cytomegalovirus) retinitis, an infection of the back of the eye that can damage the visual field severely. In its worst forms, CMV retinitis can lead to blindness, but it can be arrested with medications. This is why you should see the doctor for any visual change, and you should see him or her promptly about a rapid or asymmetric visual change.

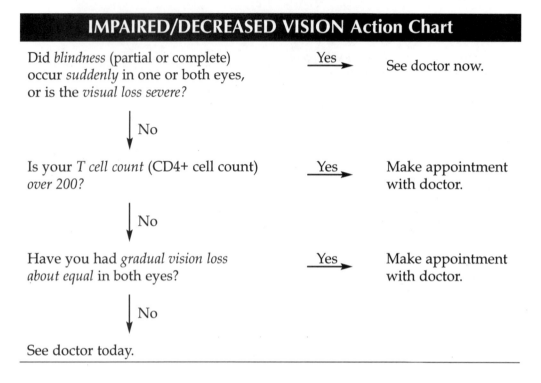

IMPAIRED/DECREASED VISION Action Chart

Did *blindness* (partial or complete) occur *suddenly* in one or both eyes, or is the *visual loss severe?* — Yes → See doctor now.

No ↓

Is your *T cell count* (CD4+ cell count) *over 200?* — Yes → Make appointment with doctor.

No ↓

Have you had *gradual vision loss about equal* in both eyes? — Yes → Make appointment with doctor.

No ↓

See doctor today.

Home Treatment of Impaired/Decreased Vision

If you experience temporary changes in your vision caused by medications or fatigue, try resting with your eyes closed in a darkened room for a few minutes. On bright days, be sure to protect your eyes with sunglasses; this will decrease strain and allow your eyes to accommodate more easily. Permanent changes in your vision should be discussed with your doctor.

Nausea and Vomiting

Many of the concerns with nausea and vomiting are the same as those with diarrhea (see page 89). Medications are the most common cause of nausea in people with HIV/AIDS, although viral infections can also cause problems. *Dehydration* is the greatest risk; as with diarrhea, intravenous medicines may be needed when it gets severe. People with severe dehydration often experience dizziness, severe thirst, dry mouth and tongue, decreased amounts of urine, dark urine, and wrin-

NAUSEA AND VOMITING Action Chart

Are *any* of the following present?
- *black or bloody vomit*
- *severe, steady abdominal pain*
- *headache and stiff neck*

→ Yes → See doctor now.

↓ No

Do you have any signs of dehydration?
- *extreme thirst*   • *very dry mouth*
- *dark urine*   • *lightheadedness*

→ Yes → See doctor now.

↓ No

Did this begin after starting a *new medication?*

→ Yes → Call doctor.

↓ No

Are you *pregnant,* or do you think you might be pregnant?

→ Yes → Call doctor.

↓ No

Have you been *vomiting* longer than 3 days without improvement?

→ Yes → Call doctor.

↓ No

Home treatment (see page 96)

---

kled, dry skin. *Vomit that is bloody or black* may indicate that severe intestinal bleeding is present. This problem is particularly bad in people with liver disease. Sometimes an infection of the brain can lead to nausea and vomiting, so if you have a *headache* and a *stiff neck,* you should see your doctor right away. Women who are sexually active should always consider the possibility that their nausea is due to pregnancy. The best way to know for sure is to get a pregnancy test, either over the counter at your local drugstore or in your doctor's office.

Many medications used in HIV/AIDS care can cause nausea. The anti-HIV drugs that can cause stomach upset include zidovidune (AZT, Retrovir), didanosine (ddI, Videx), lamivudine (3TC, Epivir), nelfinavir (Viracept), ritonavir (Norvir), and amprenavir (Agenerase); but in actuality, many different medications can have this side effect. Antibiotics and anticancer drugs are other examples. If nausea begins soon after you start a *new medicine,* call the doctor.

Home Treatment of Nausea and Vomiting

The goal of home treatment of nausea is to get as much fluid as possible into your body without upsetting your stomach any further. Sip clear fluids, such as water or ginger ale. Suck on ice chips if nothing else will stay down. Don't drink too much at any one time, as this will aggravate the stomach. Add Gatorade, bouillon, soups, and Jell-O as your condition improves. If the vomiting does not go away within three days, call the doctor.

Shortness of Breath

Shortness of breath is normal during strenuous activity. But if you get "winded" at rest or with only minimal exertion, or if you wake up at night short of breath, you have a serious symptom that should be evaluated promptly by a doctor. In people with HIV/AIDS, the major concern is pneumonia, most often caused by *Pneumocystis carinii. Pneumocystis* almost always causes a dry cough and a fever, so these symptoms are very important. Everyone must have a working thermometer and know how to use it!

There are several other causes of chronic shortness of breath, including lung damage caused by previous lung infections, anemia, and smoking-induced lung disease. These are described in Chapter 8, along with some self-management techniques that may be helpful.

Home Treatment of Shortness of Breath

Several suggestions that are often helpful for people with shortness of breath are given in Chapter 8 of this book.

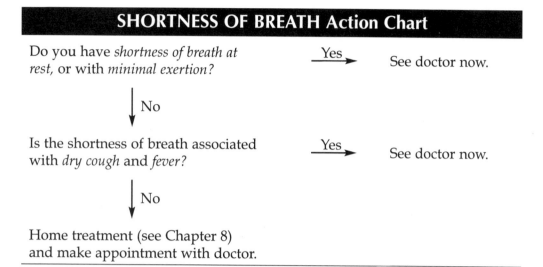

SHORTNESS OF BREATH Action Chart

Do you have *shortness of breath at rest,* or with *minimal exertion?*   → Yes → See doctor now.

↓ No

Is the shortness of breath associated with *dry cough* and *fever?*   → Yes → See doctor now.

↓ No

Home treatment (see Chapter 8) and make appointment with doctor.

Sore Throat

Sore throat is almost never a life-threatening problem, but it can be painful. Sore throats can be caused by several infections. "Cold" viruses are the most common cause and cannot be treated successfully with antibiotics; they must run their course. Mononucleosis ("mono") is a viral infection that causes a more severe, prolonged illness with painful swelling and soreness in the throat. Even though it sounds formidable, "mono" rarely causes complications and usually gets better with rest. Again, antibiotics don't help mononucleosis.

Streptococcal bacteria ("strep throat") are another common cause of sore throat. "Strep" should be treated with antibiotics in order to prevent the small chance of an abscess forming and to prevent the kidney damage that can sometimes occur. It's hard to tell when a sore throat might be "strep throat," but it's unlikely when the sore throat is a minor part of a typical cold (runny nose, stuffy ears, etc.). A high temperature, pus in the back of the throat, or swollen tonsils can be clues indicating that strep throat might be present. Sore throat in people with HIV/AIDS can also be caused by infection with candida (thrush) or by ulcers in the throat from herpes or CMV (cytomegalovirus) infections.

None of these conditions is an emergency (unless, of course, *you are unable to eat or breathe*), but it should be looked at by a doctor. Therefore, if your sore

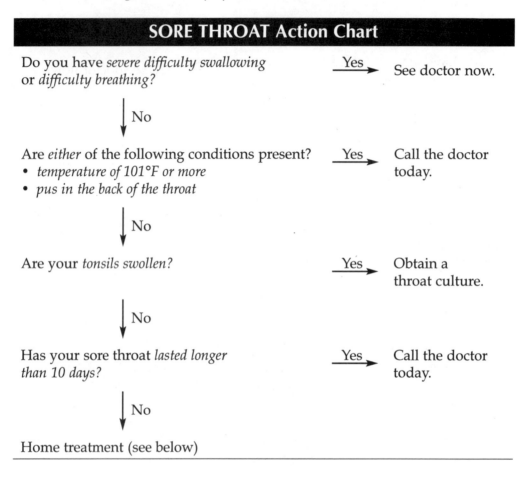

SORE THROAT Action Chart

Do you have *severe difficulty swallowing* or *difficulty breathing?* — **Yes** → See doctor now.

No

Are *either* of the following conditions present? — **Yes** → Call the doctor today.
• *temperature of 101°F or more*
• *pus in the back of the throat*

No

Are your *tonsils swollen?* — **Yes** → Obtain a throat culture.

No

Has your sore throat *lasted longer than 10 days?* — **Yes** → Call the doctor today.

No

Home treatment (see below)

throat doesn't seem to be associated with usual "cold" symptoms or if it lasts longer than ten days, you should contact your doctor.

Home Treatment of Sore Throat

Cold liquids, aspirin, ibuprofen, and acetaminophen are effective for the pain and fever. If you have had oral thrush in the past and think you might have it now (white, cottage cheese–like material in your mouth), you should start the thrush medicine your doctor gave you (usually clotrimazole [Mycelex] "troches"). Home remedies that may help include salt water gargles and honey or lemon in tea.

Urination Problems: Painful, Frequent, or Bloody Urination

Urinary infections are much more common in women than in men, but men can sometimes get them, especially if they have HIV/AIDS. The most common symptoms of urinary infection are *pain or burning on urination, frequent urgent urination,* and *blood in the urine.* But sometimes these symptoms are not caused by infection. They can also be due to excessive use of caffeine-containing beverages (coffee, tea, or cola), bladder spasms, or even anxiety. Bladder infection in women is often caused by sexual activity.

If *fever, vomiting, back pain, or teeth-chattering or body-shaking chills* are present, this suggests that the infection may have spread from the bladder to the kidneys and is much more serious. Bladder infections are common during *pregnancy,* and the treatment is more difficult. For women who get repeated bladder infections, it is important to remember to wipe the toilet tissue from front to back after urinating. Most bacteria that cause bladder infections come from the rectum.

URINATION PROBLEMS Action Chart

Are the symptoms (painful, frequent, or bloody urination) associated with fever, vomiting, back pain, or shaking chills, or is there a chance you could be *pregnant?*   —— Yes ——▶ See doctor today.

| No

Is the problem associated with a new, irritating *vaginal discharge?*   —— Yes ——▶ Is the *vaginal discharge* associated with *pain in the abdomen?*

| No | No | Yes

Home treatment (see page 100) and call the doctor today.

Home treatment (see page 100)

See doctor today.

Home Treatment of Urination Problems

Home treatment depends on drinking a lot of fluids. Drink as much as several gallons of fluid in the first twenty-four hours after symptoms start. Bacteria are literally washed out of the body with the resulting urination. Drink fruit juices to put more acid into the urine; cranberry juice is the most effective, since it contains a natural antibiotic. Begin home treatment as soon as you notice the symptoms. Relief may well begin before you see the doctor.

Sometimes irritation from the vagina can cause frequent urination or blood in the urine. When this happens, the infection may not be in the urinary system, but in the vagina or cervix. If there is *pain in the abdomen* along with *vaginal discharge,* this suggests a serious disease, ranging from gonorrhea to an ectopic pregnancy in the fallopian tube. These conditions are also suggested by *bloody discharge* that comes between periods, frequently or in large amounts. All these conditions should be evaluated by the doctor. Candida yeast (the same thing that causes thrush) often causes discharge from the vagina—it looks like white, cheesy material. It may respond to over-the-counter anti-yeast medications (Monistat, Mycolog), but some women with HIV/AIDS need stronger medicines available only by prescription.

The major concern in women with discharge from the vagina is the possibility of sexually transmitted disease (STD). All the organisms that cause STDs can cause severe infections in women with HIV/AIDS. If sexual contact in the past few weeks might possibly have led to an STD, you *must* see a doctor. It's okay to start home self-management, but make an appointment with the doctor, too.

Women who are taking antibiotics often get worse yeast infections in the vagina. To prevent these infections, it's helpful to eat yogurt, buttermilk, or sour cream and to use less sugar and alcohol. It may be helpful to call the doctor for advice on changing the medication.

Suggested Reading

Vickery, Donald M., and Fries, James F. *Take Care of Yourself.* Reading, Mass.: Addison-Wesley, 1989.

Ward, Darrell E. *The AmFAR AIDS Handbook.* New York: W.W. Norton & Company, 1999.

8

Understanding the Symptom Cycle

Being able to identify and evaluate symptoms is only part of what is necessary to become an effective self-manager. The other part is being able to understand the different causes of these symptoms, so that you can prevent them or manage them better. While it may seem as though it should be easy to identify the symptoms bothering you and what their causes are, this is not always so. People with HIV/AIDS experience many symptoms, including fatigue, stress, anger, depression, and sleeping problems. Often these symptoms are complex and interrelated, creating a vicious cycle in which one symptom feeds into another, causing more discomfort and other problems. Sometimes the symptoms and associated problems are not easily treated with medications, so it is necessary to find other ways to deal with them.

In this chapter we will discuss some of the more common symptoms that people with HIV/AIDS experience. We will look at the different factors that cause or intensify these symptoms and suggest some ways to break the vicious cycle.

Anger—Why Me?

Anger is one of the most common responses to having HIV/AIDS. The uncertainty and unpredictability of living with HIV/AIDS threatens what you have fought all your life to achieve—independence and control. The loss of control over your body and loss of independence in life create feelings of frustration, helplessness, and hopelessness, all of which fuel the anger. In fact, at various times during the course of your illness, you may find yourself asking, "Why me?" You may wonder what you did to deserve this. All of these are normal responses to HIV/AIDS.

You may be angry with yourself, your partner, family, friends, health care providers, God, or the world in general—all for a variety of reasons. You may be angry at yourself for becoming HIV infected in the first place. You may be angry at your partner, family, and friends because they don't do things the way you would like them done. You may be angry at your doctor because he or she cannot "fix" you. Other people's attitudes about you and this disease may also anger you. Sometimes your anger may be misplaced, as when you find yourself yelling at the cat or dog. Misplaced anger is quite common, especially if you are not even aware that you are angry or why.

Sometimes the anger is not just a response to having HIV/AIDS but is actually the result of the disease process itself. For example, if you have suffered an infection that has affected a certain part of the brain, your ability to express or suppress emotions may be affected. Some people who have had brain infections thus appear to cry for no reason or have flares of temper.

Recognizing (or admitting) that you are angry and identifying why, or with whom, are important in learning how to manage your anger. This task also involves finding constructive ways to express your anger. If not expressed, the anger becomes unhealthy. It can build up until it becomes explosive and offends others or is turned inward, intensifying other disease symptoms, such as depression.

Dealing with Anger

There are several things that you can do to help manage your anger:

- *Learn how to communicate your anger verbally,* preferably without blaming or offending others. (Using "I" messages rather than "you" messages to express your feelings will help you avoid blaming; these are discussed more fully in Chapter 13.) However, if you choose to express your anger verbally, know that many people will not be able to help you. Most of us are not very good at, or comfortable with, dealing with angry people, even if the anger is justified. Therefore, you may also find it useful to seek counseling or join a support group. Voluntary organizations, such as your local AIDS foundation, may have information about these.

- *Modify your expectations.* You have done this throughout your life. For example, as a child you thought you could become anything— a firefighter, a ballet dancer, a doctor. As you grew older, however, you reevaluated these expectations along with your talents and interests. From this reevaluation, you modified your plans. You can use this same process to deal with the effects of HIV/AIDS on your life. For example, it may be unrealistic to expect that you will get "all better." However, it is realistic to expect that you can still do many pleasurable things. You have the ability to affect the progress of your illness by slowing it down or preventing it from becoming worse. Changing your expectations can help you to change your perspective. Instead of dwelling on the 10 percent of things you can no longer do, think about the 90 percent of things you still can do. You may even be able to find new activities or hobbies to replace the old ones. Learning to think positively or to talk to yourself positively can also help to change your perspective. We discuss this more in Chapter 9.

- *Channel your anger through new activities,* such as exercise, writing, listening to music, and painting. Some people find these to be excellent outlets for angry feelings.

In short, anger is a normal response to having HIV/AIDS. Part of learning to manage the disease involves acknowledging this anger and finding constructive ways to deal with it.

Depression

Depression can be a frightening word. Some people prefer to say that they are "blue" or "feeling down." Whatever you call it, depression is a normal reaction to HIV/AIDS. It is not always easy to recognize when you are depressed. Even more difficult is recognizing when you may be becoming depressed and then catching yourself before you fall into a deep depression. Just as there are many degrees of pain, there are many degrees of depression. If your disease is a significant problem in your life, you almost certainly have, or have had, some problems with depression. Although depression is felt by everyone at some time, it is how you handle it that makes the difference. There are many different signs of depression, which will be discussed later in this section.

Emotions Leading to Depression

Several emotions can lead to depression:

- *Fear, anxiety, and/or uncertainty about the future.* Whether these feelings result from worries about finances, the disease process, your partner, or your family, constant worry about these issues can lead to depression if they are not addressed by you and those involved. In Chapter 15 we discuss some decisions all of us will have to make at some time in our lives. By confronting these issues early on, you will put your mind at rest and have more time to enjoy life.

- *Frustration.* A number of things can call up feelings of frustration. You may find yourself thinking, "I just can't do what I want," "I feel so helpless," "I used to be able to do this myself," or "Why doesn't anyone understand me?" Feelings like these can leave you feeling more alone and isolated the longer you hold on to them.

- *Loss of control over your life.* Whether it comes from having to rely on medications, having to see a doctor on a regular basis, or having to count on others to help you perform your daily activities—such as bathing, dressing, and preparing meals—the feeling of losing control can make you lose faith in yourself and your abilities. Your life has suddenly become a team sport in which you are no longer the coach. You are now a player with someone else calling the plays.

Although the signs of depression are listed separately, they are often experienced in combination, making it more difficult to determine what is really at the root of the depression. Also, we often do not recognize when we are depressed or do not wish to admit to ourselves that we are actually depressed. Learning to recognize the signs of depression is the first step in learning how to manage it.

Dealing with Depression

It is undeniable that having HIV/AIDS can be very depressing. We would not try to tell you that you should not have feelings of depression about your illness. However, just as the physical deconditioning resulting from HIV/AIDS can make you feel weak and helpless, leading to less physical activity and even more deconditioning, depression can be a vicious cycle of emotional "deconditioning." Depression can cause you to feel helpless and hopeless and to let go of many of your normally pleasurable activities, which in turn makes life seem even more bleak.

Depression makes us see things darkly, and from the standpoint of being depressed, we tend to believe that nothing can be changed. Not so! Depression is something that you can manage, just like any other symptom of HIV/AIDS. As part of being very depressed, however, you may not be able to dredge up

Signs of Depression

- *Loss of interest in friends or activities.* Not wanting to talk to anyone or answer the phone or doorbell.

- *Difficulty sleeping,* changed sleeping patterns, interrupted sleep, or sleeping more than usual. You may go to sleep easily but awaken often and be unable to go back to sleep.

- *Changes in eating habits.* This may range from a loss of interest in food to unusually erratic or excessive eating.

- *Unintentional weight change,* either gain or loss, of more than 10 pounds in a short period of time.

- *Loss of interest in personal care and grooming.*

- *A general feeling of unhappiness* lasting longer than 6 weeks.

- *Loss of interest in being held or in sex.* These problems can sometimes be due to medication side effects, so it is important that you talk them over with your doctor.

- *Suicidal thoughts.* If your unhappiness has caused you to think about killing yourself, get some help from your doctor, good friends, a member of the clergy, a psychologist, or a social worker. These feelings will pass and you will feel better, so get help and don't let a tragedy happen to you and your loved ones.

- *Frequent accidents.* Watch for a pattern of increased carelessness, accidents while walking or driving, dropping things, and so forth. Of course you must take into account how much the physical problems caused by your disease, such as unsteady balance or slowed reaction time, may be contributing to these incidents.

- *Poor self-image or low self-esteem.* A feeling of worthlessness, a negative image of your body, wondering if it is all worth it.

- *Frequent arguments.* A tendency to blow up easily over minor matters, things that never bothered you before.

- *Loss of energy.* Feeling tired all the time.

- *Inability to make decisions.* Feeling confused and unable to concentrate.

the motivation to get started. You may need to force yourself into action or get someone to help you do the things that will help.

Here are some active steps you can take to manage depression:

- *Seek help immediately if you feel like hurting yourself or someone else.* Call your mental health center, doctor, suicide prevention center, a friend, spiritual counselor, or community center. Do not delay. Do it now. Often, just talking with an understanding person or health professional will be enough to help you through this mood.

- *Discontinue tranquilizers or narcotic painkillers,* such as Valium, Librium, codeine, Vicodin, sleeping medications, or other downers. These drugs intensify depression, and the sooner you can stop taking them, the better off you will be. Your depression may be a drug side effect. If you are not sure what you are taking or are uncertain if what you're experiencing could be a side effect, check with a doctor or pharmacist. However, before discontinuing a prescription medication, *always* check, at least by phone, with the prescribing physician. There may be important reasons to keep taking the medicine, or there may be withdrawal reactions.

- *Cut back on drinking alcohol.* Although you may be drinking to feel better, alcohol is also a downer. There is virtually no way to escape depression unless you unload your brain of chemical downers such as alcohol. For most people, one or two drinks in the evening is not a problem, but if your mind is not free of alcohol during most of the day, you are having trouble with this drug.

- *Continue your daily activities.* Get dressed every day, make your bed, get out of the house, go shopping, walk your dog. Plan and cook meals. Force yourself to do these things even if you don't feel like it.

- *Visit with friends.* Call them on the phone. Plan to go to the movies or on other outings. Do it!

- *Join a group.* Get involved in a church group, a discussion group, a community college class, a self-help class, or a nutrition program.

- *Volunteer.* People who help other people are seldom depressed.

- *Make plans and carry them out.* Look to the future. Plant some young trees. Look forward to some special occasion. If you know that one time of the year is especially difficult, such as Christmas or a birthday, make specific plans for that period. Don't wait to see what happens. Be prepared.

- *Don't move to a new setting* without first visiting for a few weeks. Moving can be a sign of withdrawal, and depression often intensifies when you are in a location away from friends and acquaintances. Troubles usually move with you.

- *Take a vacation* with relatives or friends. Vacations can be as simple as a few days in a nearby city or in a resort just a few miles down the road. Rather than go alone, look into trips sponsored by colleges, city recreation departments, the "Y," clubs, support groups, or church groups.

- *Do twenty to thirty minutes of physical exercise every day.*

- *Make a list of self-rewards.* You can reward yourself by doing something special for yourself, such as reading at a set time or seeing a play. Anything, big or small, that you can look forward to during the day can help combat feelings of depression.

- *If you are very depressed, talk to your doctor or nurse about taking an antidepressant medication.* Such drugs can be very helpful, and one of them may be appropriate for you.

Depression feeds on depression, so *break the cycle.* The success of your self-management program depends on it. Depression is not permanent, and you can hasten its disappearance. Focus on your pride, your friends, your goals, and your positive surroundings. How you respond to depression is a self-fulfilling prophecy. When you believe that things will get better, they will.

Fatigue

HIV/AIDS can drain your energy. For many people, fatigue is a very real problem and not "all in the mind." It can keep you from doing the things you'd like to do. Furthermore, the effects of fatigue may be misunderstood or underestimated by others. Sometimes family, friends, and partners do not understand the unpredictability of the fatigue associated with HIV/AIDS and may misinterpret it as being a lack of interest in certain activities or a desire to be alone.

Fatigue can have many causes, including these:

- *The disease itself.* When you have HIV/AIDS, activities require more energy. The body is less efficient because some of the energy usually reserved for daily activities is now needed to help the body heal itself.

- *Inactivity.* Muscles that aren't used become deconditioned; that is, they become less efficient at doing what they are supposed to do. The heart, which is made of muscular tissue, can also become deconditioned. When this happens, the heart's ability to pump blood, nutrients, and oxygen to other parts of the body is decreased. When muscles do not receive the nutrients and oxygen they need to function properly, they tire more easily than muscles in good condition—the ones that receive an adequate supply of blood, oxygen, and nutrients through physical activity.

- *Poor nutrition.* Food is your basic source of energy. If the fuel you take in is not of top quality and/or in proper quantities, fatigue can result.

- *Insufficient rest.* For a variety of reasons, there will be times when you do not get enough sleep or have poor-quality sleep. This can also result in fatigue. The final section of this chapter deals with sleep problems.

- *Emotions.* Stress and depression can also cause fatigue. Most people are aware of the connection between stress and feeling tired, but fatigue is also an important symptom of depression.

  If fatigue is a problem for you, your first job is to *determine the cause.*

- Are you *exercising?*

- Are you *eating well?*

- Are you getting enough good-quality *sleep?*

If you answer no to any of these questions, you may be well on the way to determining the reasons for your fatigue. The important thing to remember about your fatigue is that it may be caused by many things other than your illness. Therefore, in order to fight and prevent fatigue, you must address the cause(s).

People often say they can't exercise because they feel fatigued. This creates a vicious cycle: you are fatigued because of a lack of exercise, and then you don't exercise because of the fatigue. Believe it or not, if this is your problem, then motivating yourself to do a little *exercise* next time you are fatigued may be the answer. You don't have to run a marathon; just go outdoors and take a short walk. If this is not possible, then walk around your house. See Chapter 10 for more information on getting started on an exercise program.

If your fatigue is caused by eating too many empty calories in the form of junk food or alcohol, the solution is to eat better-quality food as well as proper quantities of food. For some people, the problem may be a decreased interest in food, leading to not eating enough and subsequent weight loss. Other people may not absorb food well due to GI tract problems. Chapters 11 and 12 discuss in greater detail some of the problems associated with eating poorly and offer tips for improving your eating habits.

If you are having trouble getting to sleep, getting enough sleep, or staying asleep during the night, then it is very likely that your body is not getting the time it needs to replenish its energy. This can lead to fatigue. We offer some suggestions to help you get a better night's sleep later in this chapter.

If *emotions* are causing your fatigue, rest will not help; in fact, it may make you feel worse. We know that *fatigue is often a sign of depression,* and we discussed ways to deal with depression earlier in this chapter. *Stress* can also cause fatigue; at the end of this chapter, we suggest ways to manage it.

Pain

Pain is a problem shared by many people with HIV/AIDS. In fact, it may be their number one concern. As with most symptoms, pain can have many causes.

Common Causes

The four most common causes of pain are the following:

- *The disease itself.* Pain can come from damaged nerves, swollen internal organs, or irritated skin, just to name a few.

- *Tense muscles.* When something hurts, the muscles in that area become tense. This is your body's natural reaction to pain—to try to protect the damaged area.

- *Muscle deconditioning.* It is common for people with HIV/AIDS to become less active, leading to a weakening of the muscles, or muscle deconditioning. When a muscle is weak, it tends to complain anytime it is used. Thus, even the slightest activity can sometimes lead to pain and stiffness.

- *Fear and depression.* When you are afraid, frustrated, or depressed, everything, including pain, seems worse. This is not to imply that the pain is not real. Rather, fear and depression tend to make an already bad experience worse.

Because pain comes from many sources, pain management must be aimed at all of those that apply. Medications can help with some disease-caused pain; for example, they can help open blood vessels and bronchial tubes or reduce pain caused by inflammation.

Dealing with Pain

Two of the best ways of dealing with pain are *exercise* and *cognitive pain management* techniques, such as relaxation and visualization, in which you actively use your mind to help manage your symptoms. The benefits of exercise, as well as tips for starting an exercise program, are discussed in Chapter 10; using your mind to manage symptoms is discussed in Chapter 9.

In addition to exercise and cognitive pain management, several other techniques, such as *heat, cold,* and *massage,* are sometimes useful for localized pain. These three methods work by stimulating the skin and other tissues surrounding the painful area, which increases the blood flow to the area.

- *Heat.* You can stimulate the blood flow by applying a heating pad or by taking a warm bath or shower (with the water flow directed at the painful area). Limit the application to fifteen or twenty minutes at a time.

- *Cold.* Some people prefer cold for soothing the pain. A bag of frozen peas or corn makes an inexpensive, reusable cold pack. Limit the application to fifteen or twenty minutes at a time.

- *Massage* is actually one of the oldest forms of pain management. Hippocrates (c. 460–380 B.C.) said that "physicians must be experienced in many things, but assuredly also in the rubbing that can bind a joint that is loose and loosen a joint that is too hard." Self-massage is a simple method that you can use with little practice or preparation. It stimulates the skin, underlying tissues, and muscles by means of applying pressure. Some people like to use a mentholated cream with self-massage because it gives a cooling effect. Massage, however, is not appropriate for all cases of pain. Do *not* use self-massage for a "hot joint" (one that is red, swollen, and hot to the touch) or an infected area, or if you are suffering from phlebitis, thrombophlebitis, or skin eruptions. For more details on specific types of massage, see the "Suggested Reading" list at the end of this chapter.

Shortness of Breath

Shortness of breath can be a chronic symptom, or it can be caused by an acute infection that could be dangerous if not cleared up with proper treatment. To rule out the possibility of an acute infection, be sure to check your symptoms against the Shortness of Breath action chart in Chapter 7 before going on to the things discussed in this section. Shortness of breath, like fatigue and stress, can have many causes. In all cases, your body is not getting the oxygen that it needs. The difference comes in the physiological changes taking place as the result of HIV/AIDS that may lead to an increased sensitivity to different stimuli.

Common Causes

Here are some of the most common physiological changes that take place as a result of HIV/AIDS and that lead to shortness of breath:

- *Damage to the air sacs* in the lungs, as is the result of some lung infections. Such damage causes the lungs to be less efficient at getting oxygen into the blood and carbon dioxide out. Although the body can adjust to this change to some extent, when there is a sudden change in your "normal" breathing pattern the lungs cannot always keep up.

- *Narrowing of the airways to the air sacs* and *excess mucus production.* Because the airways become narrowed, there is less room for air to flow through to get to the lungs. Excess mucus production also decreases the amount of space available for oxygen to get to the lungs. These changes occur with both asthma and chronic bronchitis.

- *Anemia.* Oxygen is carried in the red blood cells, so people who are anemic (have too few red blood cells) may develop shortness of breath.

- *Deconditioning of muscles.* The deconditioning process can affect the breathing muscles or any of the other muscles in your body. When muscles become deconditioned, they are less efficient in doing what they are supposed to do, so they require more energy (and oxygen) to perform their activities. In the case of the breathing muscles, the process of clearing the lungs becomes less efficient, and less space is left for fresh air to be inhaled.

- *Anxiety and stress.* Anxiety can speed up your breathing and make it difficult to take full, deep breaths.

Dealing with Shortness of Breath

Just as there are many causes of shortness of breath, there are many things that you can do to manage this problem.

- *Don't stop what you are doing or hurry up to finish* when you feel short of breath. Instead, *slow down*. If shortness of breath continues, stop for a few minutes. If you are still short of breath, take medication if it has been prescribed by your doctor. Often shortness of breath is frightening, and this fear can cause two additional problems. First, fear can cause the body to release hormones that may cause more shortness of breath. Second, fear may cause you to stop your activity and thus never build up the endurance necessary to help your breathing. The basic rule is to take things slowly and in steps.

- *Increase your activity level gradually,* generally not by more than 25 percent each week. Thus, if you are now able to garden comfortably for twenty minutes, next week increase your time by a maximum of five minutes. Once you can garden comfortably for twenty-five minutes, you can again add a few more minutes.

- *Don't smoke.* If you are a smoker, this is easier said than done. Most smokers are addicted to smoking and nicotine without realizing it. When you try to quit, the unpleasant symptoms of withdrawal, such as lightheadedness, sleepiness, and headaches, make it very difficult. These symptoms subside in a few weeks but can still leave you with a craving for nicotine. Your doctor can prescribe a nicotine patch or gum to help you through the process of withdrawal. Another alternative is to find ways to distract or occupy yourself until the urge to smoke passes, such as chewing gum, walking around for a few minutes, brushing your teeth, or calling a friend. With time, the urges become less frequent.

  In addition to getting over the addiction to nicotine, you may find that you miss the physical motions associated with smoking. Try to find something else to keep your hands busy. You may also need to distract yourself or learn to substitute another activity for smoking when you are drinking coffee, finishing meals, reading, or watching television.

  For some, it is the fear of failing that keeps them from even trying to quit. Whatever your reasons or difficulties are, however, there are many resources that can help you when you decide to quit, such as the American Cancer Society, the American Heart

Association, the American Lung Association, your local community hospital or health maintenance organization, and the health department. Many of these organizations offer courses or materials to help you stop smoking on your own or in a group setting.

- *Avoid the smoke of others.* Avoiding "secondhand smoke" is as important in managing shortness of breath as stopping smoking. This may sometimes be hard to do because smoking friends do not realize how difficult they are making your life. Your job is to tell them. Explain that their smoke is causing breathing problems for you, and you would appreciate it if they would not smoke when you are around. Make your house a "No Smoking" zone. Ask people to smoke outside.

- *Use your medications and oxygen as prescribed by your doctor.* We are constantly bombarded with messages that drugs are bad and not to be used. In many cases, this is correct. However, when you have a chronic disease, drugs can be life savers. Don't try to skimp, cut down, or go without. At the same time, more is not better, so don't take more than the prescribed amount of medication(s). Drugs, taken as prescribed, can make all the difference. This may mean using medications even when you are not having symptoms. It also means resisting the temptation to take more of the medication if the prescribed amount does not seem to be working. If you have questions about your medications or feel as if they are not working for you, discuss these concerns with your doctor *before* you stop taking the medication or start taking more than has been prescribed. Preventing a problem before it starts is much better than having to manage the problem later.

- *Drink plenty of fluids* if mucus is a problem, unless your doctor has advised you to restrict your fluid intake. The extra fluids will help to thin the mucus and make it easier to cough up. Using a humidifier may also be helpful.

- *Practice pursed-lip and diaphragmatic breathing.** As mentioned earlier, one of the problems that causes shortness of breath is a deconditioning of the diaphragm and breathing muscles. When this

---

*The material on pursed-lip and diaphragmatic breathing was taken from Thomas L. Petty, M.D., Brian Tiep, M.D., and Mary Burns, R.N., B.S., *Essentials of Pulmonary Rehabilitation,* Pulmonary Education and Research Foundation, P.O. Box 1133, Lomita, CA 90717-5133; American Lung Association, *Help Yourself to Better Breathing,* 1989.

deconditioning occurs, the lungs are not able to empty properly, leaving less room for fresh air. Practiced together, pursed-lip and diaphragmatic breathing can help strengthen and improve the coordination and efficiency of the breathing muscles, as well as decrease the amount of energy needed to breathe. In addition, these two breathing exercises can be used with any of the techniques that use the power of your mind to manage your symptoms (often referred to as cognitive symptom management techniques and described in Chapter 9) or alone, to achieve a state of relaxation.

Diaphragmatic breathing requires a little more practice to master than pursed-lip breathing. Whereas pursed-lip breathing helps you to empty the lungs of

Pursed-Lip Breathing

Use this technique during exercise or anytime you feel short of breath.

1. *Breathe in through your nose.* This may be easier if you lean forward slightly.
2. *Hold your breath* briefly.
3. *With your lips pursed* as if you were going to whistle, *breathe out slowly* through your lips. Exhaling should take twice as long as inhaling.
4. *Practice this technique for 5 to 10 minutes,* two to four times a day.

Diaphragmatic Breathing

Use this technique to strengthen your breathing muscles.

1. *Lie on your back* with pillows under your head and knees.
2. Place *one hand on your stomach* (at the base of your breastbone) and the *other hand on your upper chest.*
3. *Inhale slowly through your nose,* allowing your stomach to expand outward. Imagine that your lungs are filling with fresh air. The hand on your stomach should move upward, and the hand on your chest should not move.
4. *Breathe out slowly, through pursed lips.* At the same time, use your hand to gently push inward and upward on your abdomen.
5. *Practice this technique for 10 to 15 minutes,* three or four times a day, until it becomes automatic. If you begin to feel a little dizzy, rest.

trapped air and reestablish a normal breathing pattern, diaphragmatic breathing strengthens the breathing muscles. Strengthening these muscles makes them more efficient so that less effort is needed to breathe.

Once you feel comfortable doing diaphragmatic breathing, you may wish to place a light weight on your abdomen. This will further strengthen the muscles you use to inhale. Start with a weight of about one pound, such as a book or a bag of rice or beans. Gradually increase the weight as your muscle strength improves. Once you can breathe easily lying down, you can practice diaphragmatic breathing while sitting, while standing, and finally while walking. By mastering this technique while doing other activities, you will be better able to manage your shortness of breath.

Sleeping Problems

Sleep is the time during which the body can concentrate on healing, because little energy is required to maintain body functioning when we sleep. When we do not get enough sleep, we may experience a variety of other symptoms, such as fatigue and lack of concentration. This does not mean that fatigue or lack of concentration is always caused by a lack of sleep; remember, the symptoms associated with HIV/AIDS can have many causes. However, if you have noticed a change in your sleep patterns, then the fatigue you are experiencing may, at least in part, be related to your problems with sleep.

Dealing with Sleep Problems

Many people feel powerless to solve their sleep problems, but there are many things you can do to help yourself get a good night's sleep. To sleep well, you need to (1) have a good, comfortable place to sleep; (2) avoid putting substances in your body that interfere with sleep; (3) get into a sleep routine; and (4) learn to deal with things that might interrupt your sleep. Each of these items is covered below.

Before you even get into bed

- *Get a comfortable bed* that allows you to move around easily and provides good support. This usually means a good-quality, firm mattress that supports the spine and does not cause you to roll to the middle of the bed. A bed board, made of half-inch to three-quarter-inch plywood, can be placed between the mattress and the box spring to increase the firmness. Heated waterbeds or airbeds are helpful for some people because they support weight evenly by conforming to the body's shape. Other people find them to be very uncomfortable. If you are interested, try one out at a friend's home or a hotel for a few nights to decide if it is right for you.

- *Elevate the head of your bed* on wooden blocks 4 to 6 inches thick to make breathing easier. You can get the same effect by using pillows that elevate your chest, shoulders, and head.

- *Keep the room at a comfortable, warm temperature.*

- *Use a vaporizer* if you live where the air is dry, or in cold weather when your heating system lowers the humidity of the air in your house. Warm, moist air often makes breathing easier, leaving you with one less thing to worry about when trying to fall asleep.

- *Make your bedroom a place in which you feel safe and comfortable.* Keep a lamp and telephone by your bed within easy reach.

- *Keep a pair of glasses by the bed* if you wear glasses or contact lenses. This way, in case you need to get up in the middle of the night, you can easily put on your glasses and see where you are going!

Things to avoid before bedtime

- *Avoid eating before bedtime.* Although you may feel sleepy after a big meal, eating is no way to help you fall asleep and get a good night's rest. Sleep is supposed to allow your body time to rest and recover; but when you eat, your body is kept busy with digestion, taking valuable time away from this healing process. Since going to sleep feeling hungry may also keep you awake, try drinking a glass of warm milk.

- *Avoid alcohol.* Contrary to the belief that alcohol will help you to sleep better because it makes you feel more relaxed, alcohol actually disrupts your sleep cycle. Alcohol before bedtime can lead to shallow and fragmented sleep, as well as frequent awakenings throughout the night.

- *Avoid caffeine late in the day.* Because caffeine is a stimulant, it can keep you awake. Caffeine is found not only in coffee, but also in some types of teas, colas and other sodas, and chocolate.

- *Avoid eating foods with MSG (monosodium glutamate) late in the day.* Although Chinese foods are often singled out as containing MSG, many other types of food, especially prepackaged foods, may contain this food additive. Before purchasing a prepackaged meal, be sure to read the ingredient label to check that the food does not contain monosodium glutamate.

- *Don't smoke to help you sleep.* The nicotine in cigarettes is a stimulant. And aside from the fact that smoking itself can cause complications and worsening of lung problems, falling asleep with a lit cigarette is a fire hazard.

- *Avoid diet pills.* Diet pills often contain stimulants that may interfere with falling asleep as well as staying asleep.

- *Avoid sleeping pills.* Although sleeping pills sound like the perfect solution to sleep problems, they tend to become less effective over time. Also, many sleeping pills have a rebound effect—that is, if you stop taking them, it becomes more difficult to get to sleep. You may end up having even more problems than you had when you first started taking the sleeping pills. It is best to avoid using sleeping pills if at all possible.

Developing a routine

- *Set up a regular rest and sleep pattern.* Go to bed at the same time every night and get up at the same time every morning. If you wish to take a nap, take one in the afternoon, but do not take a nap after dinner. Stay awake until you are ready to go to bed.

- *Reset your sleep clock if your sleep pattern is way off the norm* (for example, if you go to bed at 4:00 A.M. and sleep until noon). To do so, try going to bed one hour earlier or later each day until you reach the hour you want to go to bed. This method may seem strange, but it seems to be the best way to reset your sleep clock.

- *Exercise at regular times each day.* Not only will the exercise help you have better-quality sleep, exercising at the same time every day will also help to set a regular pattern for your day.

- *Get out in the sun every afternoon,* even if it is only for fifteen or twenty minutes. The sun is necessary to keep your "body clock" correctly set.

- Get used to doing the *same things every night before going to bed*. This can be anything from watching the news, to reading a chapter of a book, to taking a warm bath. By developing and sticking to a getting-ready-for-bed routine, you will be telling your body that it's time to start winding down and relax.

But I can't fall (back) asleep

- *Use your bed and your bedroom only for sleeping and for sex.* If you get into bed and find that you can't fall asleep, get out of bed and go into another room until you begin to feel sleepy again.
- *Don't keep a TV set in the bedroom.* Often people have a TV set in the bedroom, thinking that it helps them fall asleep. It doesn't. It actually keeps the mind racing and interferes with sleep. You might think, "But I always fall asleep with the TV on!" But do you ever fall asleep *early* with it on? Not likely. Probably it's sometime during the late show!
- *Refocus your mind away from worries.* You may get to sleep without a problem but then wake up with the "early morning worries," in which you can't turn off your mind. Then you get more worried because you cannot go back to sleep once you have awakened. Keeping your mind occupied with something else will ward off the worries and help you get back to sleep. For example, try quieting your mind by counting backward from 100 by threes or naming a flower for every letter of the alphabet.
- *Don't worry about not getting enough sleep.* If your body needs sleep, you will sleep. Also, remember that people tend to need less sleep as they get older.

Stress

Stress is a common problem for everyone. But what *is* stress? In the 1950s, physiologist Hans Selye described stress as "the nonspecific response of the body to any demand made upon it." Others have expanded this definition to define stress as the body's adaptation to demands, whether pleasant or unpleasant.

How Does Your Body Respond to Stress?

Your body is used to functioning at a certain level. When there is a need to change this level, your body must adjust physiologically to meet the demand. Your body reacts by preparing itself to take an action: your heart rate increases, your blood pressure rises, your neck and shoulder muscles tense, your breathing becomes more rapid, your digestion slows, your mouth becomes dry, and you may begin sweating. These are typical signals of stress.

What causes stress responses?

To take an action, your muscles need a supply of oxygen and energy. Your rate of breathing increases in an effort to inhale as much oxygen as possible and to get rid of as much carbon dioxide as possible. Your heart rate increases to deliver the oxygen and nutrients to the muscles.

How long will the stress responses last?

In general, stress responses are present only until the stressful event passes. Your body then returns to its normal level of functioning. Sometimes, though, your body does not return to its former comfortable level. If the stress is present for any length of time, your body begins adapting to this stress. This adaptation can contribute to the development of health problems such as hypertension (high blood pressure) and shortness of breath.

Common Types of Stressors

Regardless of the type of stressor (the thing that causes a stress response), the changes in the body are the same. Stressors, however, are not completely independent of one another. In fact, one stressor can often lead to other types of stressors or even magnify existing stressors. Several stressors can also occur at the same time. This works in much the same way as the vicious cycle of deconditioning and helplessness described in Chapter 1.

These are some of the more common sources and types of stress:

- *Physical stressors.* Physical stressors can range from something as pleasant as going out dancing, to grocery shopping, to something unpleasant, like the physical symptoms of your HIV/AIDS. The one thing that these three stressors have in common is that they all increase your body's demand for energy. If your body is not prepared to deal with this demand, the results may be sore muscles, fatigue, and a worsening of some disease symptoms.

- *Mental and emotional stressors.* Mental and emotional stressors can range from pleasant to uncomfortable. The joys you experience in seeing your sister get married or meeting new friends induce the same stress response in the body as feeling frustrated or down because of your illness. Although it seems strange that this is true, the difference comes in the way the stress is perceived by your brain.

- *Environmental stressors.* Environmental stressors can also be good or bad. They may be as varied as a sunny day, uneven sidewalks that make it difficult to walk, loud noises, and secondhand smoke.

Recognizing When You Feel Stressed

In reality, you have a certain need for stress—it helps your life run more efficiently. As long as you don't go past your breaking point, stress is helpful. On some days you can tolerate more stress than on others. But sometimes, if you are not aware of the different types of stress you are experiencing, you can go beyond your breaking point and feel like your life is completely out of control. It is often difficult to recognize when you are under too much stress.

The warning signs of stress include:

- biting your nails, pulling your hair, or other repetitive habits
- grinding your teeth, clenching your jaw
- tension in your head, neck, or shoulders (which can cause headaches)
- feelings of anxiousness, nervousness, helplessness, or irritability

Sometimes you can catch yourself engaging in these stress responses. If you do, take a few minutes to think about what it is that is making you feel tense. Take a few deep breaths and try to relax. Some methods for using your mind to help you relax are presented in Chapter 9.

Dealing with Stress

Stress can't be "cured," because it's part and parcel of everyday life. But you can learn to deal with the bad effects of stress. Two ways of coping with stress are (1) *avoiding* stressful situations and (2) *managing* stressful situations.

Avoiding Stressful Situations

Some situations are immediately identifiable as stressful—for example, being stuck in traffic, going on a trip, preparing meals, or going on a job interview. First, *look, as objectively as possible, at what it is about the particular situation that is stressful.* Is it that you hate to be late? Are trips stressful because of the uncertainty involved with your destination? Does meal preparation involve too many steps that demand too much energy?

Once you have determined what specifically is stressful about a situation, you can *begin looking for ways to avoid the aspects of the situation that are creating stress for you.* Can you leave earlier? Can you let someone else drive? Can you call someone at your destination site and ask about wheelchair access, local mass transit, and so on? Can you prepare food in the morning? Can you take a short nap in the early afternoon? After you have identified some possible solutions, *select one* to try the next time you are in this situation. Don't forget to *evaluate the results.* (This is the problem-solving approach we discussed in Chapter 2.)

Managing the Stress

Although you can successfully manage some types of stress by avoiding the stressful parts of the situation, many other types of stress seem to sneak up on you when you don't expect them. Dealing with this type of stress also involves the problem-solving approach.

If you know that certain situations will be stressful, *develop ways to deal with them before they happen.* Try to *rehearse,* in your mind, what you will do when the situation arises. Inherent in this approach is listening to your body for signals that the tension and stress are building. The better you become at listening and understanding your body's signals, the better you'll become at managing your stress and stressful situations.

Certain chemicals, such as nicotine, alcohol, and caffeine, can also increase stress. Although you may smoke a cigarette, drink a glass of wine, or drink a cup of coffee to soothe your tension, these substances, in fact, actually increase the stress response in your body. Eliminating these stressors can leave you feeling calmer.

Chapter 9, "Using Your Mind to Manage Symptoms," discusses mental techniques, such as self-talk, progressive muscle relaxation, guided imagery, and visualization, that may also be useful to you in stressful situations. Other ways to deal with stress, such as getting enough sleep, exercising, and eating well, are discussed in this chapter and in Chapters 10 and 11.

In summary, stress, like every other symptom, has many causes and, therefore, has more than one way to be managed. It is up to you to examine the problem and try those solutions that meet your needs and lifestyle.

Taking actions to physically deal with your symptoms is necessary in coping with your illness on a day-to-day basis. But sometimes this just doesn't seem to be enough. There are times during the day when you may wish to escape from your surroundings and just have "your time"—a time that allows you to clear your mind, to gain a fresh perspective. The following chapter will show you different ways to complement your physical symptom management with *cognitive techniques*—techniques in which you use your mind to help reduce and even prevent some of the symptoms commonly experienced with HIV/AIDS.

Suggested Reading

Ball, Nigel, and Hough, Nick. *The Sleep Solution: A 21-Night Program for Restful Sleep*. Berkeley: Ulysses Press, 1988.

Carter, Les, and Minirth, Frank. *The Anger Workbook: A 13-Step Interactive Plan*. Nashville: Thomas Nelson, 1993.

Caudill, Margaret A., *Managing Pain Before It Manages You*. New York: Guilford Press, 1995.

Cooper, Kenneth H. *Can Stress Help? Converting a Major Health Hazard into a Surprising Benefit*. Nashville: Thomas Nelson, 1997.

Cunningham, J. Barton, and Cunningham, Bart. *The Stress Management Sourcebook: Everything You Need to Know*. Chicago: Contemporary Publishing, 1997.

Falten, Sharon, and Diamond, D. *Tension Turnaround: The 30-Day Program for Inner Calm, Confidence and Control*. Emmaus, Penn.: Rodale Press, 1990.

Johnson, T. Scott, and Halberstadt, Jerry. *Phantom of the Night*. Cambridge: New Technology, 1995.

Kabat-Zinn, Jon. *Full Catastrophe Living: Using the Wisdom of Your Body and Mind to Face Stress, Pain and Illness*. New York: Delta, 1996.

Kleinke, Chris L. *Coping with Life Changes*. 2nd ed. Pacific Grove, Calif: Brooks/Cole, 1997.

Lewinsohn, Peter, with Munoz, Ricardo, Youngren, Mary, and Zeiss, Antoinette. *Control Your Depression*. Englewood Cliffs, N.J.: Prentice Hall, 1987.

Natelson, Benjamin H. *Facing and Fighting Fatigue: A Practical Approach*. New Haven, Conn.: Yale University Press, 1998.

Powell, Trevor. *Free Yourself from Harmful Stress*. Chesham, England: Dorley Kindersley Ltd., 1997.

Seidman, David. *The Longevity Source Book*. Los Angeles: Lowell House, 1997.

Shone, Neville. *Coping Successfully with Pain*. Boston: G.K. Hall & Co., 1993.

Zammit, Gary. *Good Nights: How to Stop Sleep Deprivation, Overcome Insomnia and Get the Sleep You Need*. Kansas City, Mo.: Andrews & McMeel, 1997.

Using Your Mind to Manage Symptoms

All of us, at one time or another, have experienced the power of the mind and its effects on the body. Our thoughts and feelings, both pleasant and unpleasant, can cause the body to react in different ways. Often the heart rate and breathing are affected. We may also experience other sensations such as perspiration, warm or cold; blushing; or tears. Sometimes just a memory or image can create these responses. For example, take a moment now and think about a big, juicy lemon. Now think about sucking on the lemon. What happens? Your mouth puckers and starts to water. You may even smell the scent of the lemon. All of these reactions are triggered by the mind and its memory of a lemon.

This example demonstrates the power of the mind over the body and why it pays to develop our mental abilities to help us manage the different symptoms of HIV/AIDS. Through training and practice, we can learn to use the mind to relax the body, to reduce stress, and to decrease the discomfort caused by physical and emotional symptoms. The mind can also help to relieve pain and shortness of breath, and may even help you to depend less on medications to relieve your symptoms.

In this chapter we will describe several ways, called *cognitive techniques,* in which you can use your mind to manage symptoms.

Relaxation Techniques

Although you may have heard and read about relaxation, you may still be confused as to what it is, what its benefits are, and how to do it. Relaxation is not a cure-all, but it can be an effective part of treatment. There are different types of relaxation techniques, each with specific guidelines and uses. Some techniques are used only to achieve muscle relaxation; others are aimed at reducing anxiety and emotional arousal or at diverting attention, all of which aid in symptom management.

The term *relaxation* means different things to different people. We can all identify ways we relax. For example, we may walk, watch TV, listen to music, cook, or garden. These methods of relaxing, however, are different from the techniques discussed here because they include some form of physical activity that requires your mind's attention. Relaxation techniques are also different from taking a nap or resting because we are using the mind actively to help the body achieve a relaxed state. *The goal of relaxation is to turn off the outside world so the mind and body are at rest.* This state allows you to reduce the tension that can increase the intensity of symptoms. When you have become adept at using the relaxation techniques described here, you will find that your relaxation sessions leave you with an overall feeling of peace and well-being, as well as a lessening of your physical symptoms.

Muscle Relaxation

Muscle relaxation is one of the most commonly used cognitive techniques for symptom management. It is popular because it makes sense to us. If we are told that physical stress or muscular tension intensifies our pain, shortness of breath, or emotional distress, we are motivated to learn how to recognize this tension and release it. In addition, muscle relaxation is easy to learn and practice in different

---

Guidelines for Using Relaxation Techniques

- *Pick a quiet place and time* during the day when you will not be disturbed for at least 15–20 minutes. (If this seems too long, start with 5 minutes.)

- *Try to practice the technique twice daily,* but not less than four times a week.

- *Don't expect miracles.* Some of these techniques require time for you to acquire the skill and sometimes 3 to 4 weeks of consistent practice before you really start to notice benefits.

- *Relaxation should be helpful.* At worst, you may find it boring; but if it is an unpleasant experience or makes you more nervous or anxious, then you might try one of the other symptom management techniques described in this chapter.

situations. It is one technique in which we can recognize some immediate results, such as the positive sensations of reduced pain, stress, or muscle tension and calm, normal breathing. Muscle relaxation is not likely to fail because of distractions caused by symptoms or thoughts. It is a useful strategy to reduce pain, muscular tension, and stress while helping to control shortness of breath and to achieve a more restful sleep.

Following are two examples of muscle relaxation techniques. Try both techniques and choose the one that works best for you. Then tape-record the script for that routine. Although recording the script is not necessary, it is sometimes helpful if you find it hard to concentrate. Also, you won't be distracted by having to refer to the book when you are trying to relax.

Progressive Muscle Relaxation

Many years ago, a physiologist named Edmund Jacobson discovered that in order to relax, one must know how it feels to be tense, as well as relaxed. He believed that if one learned to recognize tension, then one could learn to let it go and relax. He designed a simple exercise to assist with this learning process.

To relax muscles, you need to know how to scan your body, recognize where you are holding tension, and release that tension. The first step is to become familiar with the difference between the feeling of *tension* and the feeling of *relaxation*. The brief progressive muscle relaxation exercise on pages 127–128 will allow you to compare those feelings and, with practice, identify and release tension anywhere in your body.

As Jacobson emphasizes in the exercise, the purpose of voluntarily tensing the muscles is to learn to recognize and locate tension in your body. You will then become aware of tension and use this same procedure to let it go. *Once you learn the technique, it will no longer be necessary to tense voluntarily; just locate the existing tension and let it go.*

For some people with a lot of pain, particularly in the joints, the Jacobson progressive muscle relaxation technique may not be appropriate. If it causes any pain, the pain may distract you from the relaxation. If this is the case, the body scan technique may work better for you.

Body Scan

The body scan is a relaxation technique similar to Jacobson's progressive muscle relaxation exercise, but it doesn't require the tensing or movement of muscle groups. Like Jacobson's exercise, it is best done while lying on your

Progressive Muscle Relaxation Exercise

This exercise guides you through the major muscle groups, asking you to first *tense* and then *relax* those muscles. If you have pain in a particular area, tense those muscles only gently or not at all and focus on relaxing them.

1. Make yourself as comfortable as possible. Loosen any clothing that feels tight. Uncross your legs and ankles. Allow your body to feel supported by the surface on which you are sitting or lying.

2. Close your eyes. Take a deep breath, filling your chest and breathing all the way down to the abdomen. Hold . . . Breathe out through pursed lips, and as you breathe out, let as much tension as possible flow out with your breath. Let all your muscles feel heavy and let your whole body just sink into the surface beneath you . . . Good.

3. Become aware of the muscles in your *feet and calves.* Pull your toes back up toward your knees. Notice the tension in your feet and calves. Release and relax. Notice the discomfort leaving as relief and warmth replace it. That's it.

4. Now tighten the muscles of your *thighs and buttocks.* Hold and feel the tension. Let go and allow the muscles to relax. The relaxed muscles feel heavy and supported by the surface upon which you are sitting or lying.

5. Tense the muscles in your *abdomen and chest.* Notice a tendency to hold your breath as you tense. Relax, and notice that it is natural to want to take a deep breath to relieve the tension in this area. Take a deep breath now, breathing all the way down to the abdomen. As you breathe out, allow all the tension to flow out with your breath.

6. Now, stretching your fingers out straight, tense your fingers and tighten your *arm muscles.* Relax. Feel the tension flowing out as the circulation returns.

7. Press your shoulder blades together, tightening the muscles in your *shoulders and neck.* This is a place where many people carry a lot of tension. Hold . . . Now, let go. Notice how the muscles feel warmer and more alive.

8. Tighten all the muscles of your *face and head.* Notice the tension, especially around your eyes and in your jaw. Now relax, allowing your jaw to become slack and your mouth to remain slightly open . . . That's right. Note the difference.

(continued)

9. Now take another deep breath, breathing all the way down to the abdomen. And, as you breathe out, allow your body to sink heavily into the surface beneath you, becoming even more deeply relaxed. Good.

10. Enjoy this comfortable feeling of relaxation . . . Remember it. With practice, you will become skilled at recognizing muscle tension and releasing it.

11. Prepare to come back to the here and now. Take three deep breaths. When you're ready, open your eyes.

---

back, but any comfortable position can be used. First, you must focus on your breathing. Spend a few minutes concentrating on each breath as it enters and leaves your body. Try directing your breath past your chest, all the way down to your abdomen. (This is diaphragmatic breathing, which is described in Chapter 8 and is an important part of all relaxation exercises.)

After three or four minutes of concentrating on your breathing, put your attention on your toes. Don't move the toes; just think about how they feel. Don't worry if you don't feel anything at all. If you find any tension there, let it go as you breathe out.

After a few moments of concentrating on your toes, move your attention to the bottoms of your feet. Again, don't move; just concentrate on any sensations you may have. Let go of any tension as you breathe out. Next, concentrate on the tops of your feet and your ankles. After a few more moments, bring your attention to your lower legs.

Continue this process, shifting your attention every few moments to another part of your body, working slowly upward to your head. If you find tension, let it go as you breathe out. If your mind starts to wander, just bring your attention back to the feelings in your body and your breathing.

This technique can also be used to help you get to sleep, because it helps to clear your mind of any worries or distracting thoughts. The key is to give your full attention to scanning your body for tension and releasing it.

Imagery and Visualization Techniques

While relaxation techniques are the most common methods used to reduce muscle tension and stress, other cognitive techniques can also be useful. Techniques such as imagery and visualization can help to reduce fear, worry, and anxiety and take your mind off the unpleasantness of your symptoms.

Guided Imagery

The guided imagery relaxation technique is like a guided daydream. It allows you to refocus your mind away from your symptoms by transporting you to another time and place. It has the added benefit of helping you to achieve deep relaxation by picturing yourself in a peaceful environment. The guided imagery script presented here can help take you on this mental stroll.

There are several ways in which you can use the guided imagery script:

- You can read the script over several times to become familiar with it. Then sit or lie down in a quiet place and try to reconstruct the scene in your mind. Each script should take ten to fifteen minutes to complete.

- You can have a family member or friend read you the script slowly, pausing for five to ten seconds wherever there is a series of dots (. . .).

- You can make a tape of the script and play it to yourself whenever it's convenient.

Visualization

Visualization, also referred to as *vivid imagery,* is similar to guided imagery. It is another way of using your imagination to picture yourself any way you want, doing things you want to do. You can practice visualization in different ways and for longer, as well as brief, periods. You can also use this relaxation technique while you are engaged in other activities.

One way to use visualization is to recall pleasant scenes from your past or to create new scenes in your mind. It allows you to create more of your own images than the guided imagery technique does. For example, try to remember every detail of a special holiday or party that made you happy. Who was there? What happened? What did you talk about? You can do the same sort of thing by remembering a vacation. In fact, visualization can be used to plan the details of some future event or to fill in the details of a pleasant fantasy. For example, how would you spend a million dollars? What would be your ideal romantic encounter? What would your ideal home or garden look like? Where would you go and what would you do on your dream vacation?

Another form of visualization involves imagining symbols that represent the discomfort or pain you feel in different parts of your body. For example, a painful joint might be red, or a tight chest might have a constricting band around it. After forming these images, you then try to change them. The red

A Walk in the Country (Guided Imagery)

- Make yourself as comfortable as possible, sitting or lying down. Loosen any constricting clothing. Uncross your arms, legs, and ankles. Allow your body to feel supported by the surface on which you are sitting or lying.

- Close your eyes.

- Take a deep breath, in through your nose, breathing all the way down to the abdomen. Hold . . . Breathe out slowly through slightly pursed lips and as you do, relax your whole body, allowing all your muscles to feel limp and heavy . . . Good.

- Scan your body for any muscle tension, starting with your head and going all the way down to your toes.

- Release any tension in your face, head, and neck by letting your jaw become slack and your head feel heavy on your shoulders. Allow your shoulders to drop heavily. Take a deep breath and relax your chest and abdomen. Allow your arms and legs to feel heavy and to sink into the surface beneath you.

- Now take a deep breath and become aware of any remaining tension in your body. As you breathe out, allow all the muscles of your body to sink heavily into the surface beneath you, becoming even more deeply relaxed . . . Good.

- Imagine yourself walking along an old country road . . . the sun is warm on your back . . . the birds are singing . . . the air is calm and fragrant.

- As you progress down the road, you come across an old gate . . . The gate creaks as you open it and go through.

- You find yourself in an overgrown garden, flowers growing where they have seeded themselves, vines climbing over a fallen tree, green grass, shade trees.

- Breathe deeply, smelling the flowers . . . listen to the birds and insects . . . feel the gentle breeze, warm against your skin.

- As you walk leisurely up a gentle slope behind the garden, you come to a wooded area where the trees become denser and the sun is filtered through the leaves. The air feels mild and a bit cooler. You become aware of the sound and fragrance of a nearby brook. You breathe deeply of the cool and fragrant air several times, and with each breath you feel more refreshed.

- Soon you come upon the brook. It is clear and clean as it tumbles over the rocks and some fallen logs. You follow the path along the brook for a ways. The path takes you out into a sunlit clearing where you discover a small and picturesque waterfall . . . There is a rainbow in the mist . . .

(continued)

- You find a comfortable place to sit for a while, a perfect niche where you can feel completely relaxed.
- You feel good as you allow yourself to just enjoy the warmth and solitude of this peaceful place.
- It is now time to return. You walk back down the path, through the cool and fragrant trees, out into the sun-drenched overgrown garden . . . one last smell of the flowers, and out the creaky gate . . .
- You leave this secret retreat for now and return down the country road. However, you know that you may visit this special place whenever you wish.
- When you are ready, take three deep breaths and open your eyes whenever you wish.

color might fade until there is no more color, or the constricting band might stretch and stretch until it falls off. Visualization is also a useful technique to help you set and accomplish your personal goals (see Chapter 2). After you write your weekly action plan, take a few minutes to imagine yourself taking a walk, doing your exercises, or taking your medications. Here you are mentally rehearsing the steps you need to take in order to carry out your action plan. Studies have shown that this technique can help people cope better with stressful situations, master skills, and accomplish personal goals. In fact, those people who have become skilled at visualization find that they can actually decrease some of the discomfort and distress associated with symptoms by changing unpleasant images to pleasant ones.

All the relaxation techniques mentioned above can be used in conjunction with pursed-lip and diaphragmatic breathing. These breathing techniques, described in Chapter 8, can help you achieve a more relaxed state and keep your mind off any potential for shortness of breath.

Other Cognitive Strategies

Other cognitive strategies, such as *distraction, self-talk, meditation,* and *reflection,* take a different approach to managing symptoms. These techniques all involve retraining your patterns of thinking so that symptoms seem less intense, less limiting, or less important.

Distraction

Because the mind has trouble focusing on more than one thing at a time, you can lessen the intensity of your symptoms by training your mind to focus on something other than your body and its sensations. This technique, called *distraction* or *attention refocusing,* is particularly helpful if you feel your symptoms are overwhelming or worry that every bodily sensation might indicate a new or worsening symptom or health problem. It is important to note that with distraction you are not ignoring the symptoms, but choosing not to dwell on them.

Distraction works best for short activities or episodes in which symptoms may be anticipated, as in the following examples:

- *Make plans for exactly what you will do after the unpleasantness passes.* For example, if you have trouble falling asleep, try making plans for some future event, being as detailed as possible.

- *Think of a person's name, a bird, a flower, or other object for every letter of the alphabet.* If you get stuck on one letter, go on to the next. (These are good distractions for physical discomfort as well as for sleep problems.)

- *Count backward* from 1,000 or 100 by threes (for example, 100, 97, 94, . . .).

- *Try to remember the words to a favorite song or the events in an old story.*

There are, of course, a million variations to these examples, all of which will help you to refocus attention away from your problem.

So far we have discussed short-term distraction strategies in which you refocus your mind *internally,* away from your symptoms to thoughts of something more pleasant. There is another kind of distraction, the distraction of action, that works well for long-term projects or for symptoms that tend to last longer, such as depression and some forms of chronic pain. In this type of distraction, the mind is focused not internally but rather *externally,* on some type of activity. If you are slightly depressed or have continuous unpleasant symptoms, find an activity that interests you, and you will find yourself distracted from the problem. This activity can be almost anything, such as gardening, cooking, reading, going to a movie, or even doing volunteer work. One of the marks of a successful self-manager is that he or she has a variety of interests and always seems to be doing something.

Self-Talk: "I Know I Can"

We talk to ourselves all the time. For example, when waking up in the morning, we think, "I really don't want to get out of bed. I'm tired and don't want to go to work today." Or at the end of an enjoyable evening we think, "Gee, that was fun. I should get out more often." These things we think or say to ourselves are called "self-talk."

All of our self-talk is learned from others and becomes a part of us as we grow up. It comes in many forms, most of which are negative. Negative self-statements usually take the form of: "I just can't do . . . ," "If only I could or didn't . . . ," "I just don't have the energy to . . . ." This type of self-talk represents the doubts and fears we have about ourselves in general and about our abilities to deal with a disease and its symptoms in particular. Unfortunately, negative self-talk can have the effect of worsening symptoms such as pain, depression, and fatigue.

Because what we learn in life influences our beliefs, attitudes, feelings, and actions, what we say to ourselves plays a major role in determining our success or failure in becoming good self-managers. Learning to make self-talk work *for* you instead of *against* you, by changing those negative statements to positive ones, will help you manage your symptoms more effectively. This change, as with any habit, requires practice.

To change negative self-talk to positive:

1. *Listen carefully to what you say* to or about *yourself,* both out loud and silently. Then write down all the negative self-talk statements. Pay special attention to the things you say during times that are particularly difficult for you. For example, what do you say to yourself when getting up in the morning with pain, while doing those exercises you don't really like, or at those times when you are feeling blue?

2. *Work on* changing *each negative statement you identified to a positive one,* and write these down. Positive statements should reflect the better you and your decision to be in control. For example, negative statements such as "I don't want to get up," "I'm too tired and I hurt," "I can't do the things I like anymore so why bother," or "I'm good for nothing" become positive messages, such as "I have the energy to get up and do the things I enjoy," "I know I can do anything I believe I can," "People like me and I feel good about myself," or "Other people need and depend on me. I'm worthwhile."

3. *Read and rehearse these positive statements,* mentally or with another person. It is this conscious repetition or memorization of positive self-talk that will help you replace those old, habitual negative statements.

4. *Practice these new statements in real situations.* This practice, along with time and patience, will help your new patterns of thinking become automatic.

Once established, positive self-talk can be one of the most powerful tools you can add to your self-management program, helping you to manage symptoms as well as to master the other skills discussed in this book.

Mindfulness Meditation

There are many types of meditation. In fact, meditation is a part of most religious or spiritual traditions. The purpose of meditation is to quiet the mind. It can also help to quiet the body. For this reason, meditation is often a useful technique for managing stress and other symptoms, such as pain, fatigue, and shortness of breath. Mindfulness meditation is one type of meditation that can be practiced by anyone. All you need to begin is a quiet place and five or more minutes. Start by sitting in a chair with your feet flat on the floor and your hands in your lap or on your knees. If you wish and are able to, you can sit on the floor with crossed legs or in a more traditional yogi position. How you sit, however, does not matter.

The essence of mindfulness meditation is to concentrate fully on your breathing. It is best if you can do diaphragmatic or belly breathing, but you do not have to take deep breaths. It is important to keep your full attention on your breathing. Breathe in slowly, hold the breath for a moment, and then breathe out slowly. At all times concentrate on your breathing.

Although this seems fairly simple, you will find that your mind easily wanders. This is called "having a monkey mind." As soon as you notice that your mind is wandering, bring your attention back to your breathing. At first you may not be able to attend your breathing for more than a minute or two. You will improve, however, with practice.

When you are doing this type of meditation, you may become very aware of your body. For example, your eye may itch or you may become uncomfortable in your sitting position. When this happens, first do nothing but pay attention to your breathing. In many cases you will find that the discomfort goes away. If it continues, scratch the itch or change your position. Pay full attention to what you are doing. With mindfulness meditation it is important to be fully aware of what you are doing at each moment!

Like all other self-management techniques, mindfulness meditation requires practice. You will not get results immediately, but if you practice for fifteen to thirty minutes a day, four or five days a week, you will find that meditation can be a great symptom management tool.

Prayer or Reflection

Over the years, many people with chronic health problems have told us that prayer or reflection has been helpful in managing both the physical and emotional symptoms of their disease. For some, these practices are forms of relaxation that help reduce tension and anxiety. For others, these activities of the mind may be a method of distraction by which they refocus their attention or separate themselves from their symptoms. Regardless of the rationale, prayer

Principles of Symptom Self-Management

- *Symptoms have many causes.* Thus, there are many ways to manage most symptoms. Understanding the nature and varied causes of your symptoms and how these interact will help you to better manage your symptoms.

- *Not all management techniques will work for everyone.* It is up to you to experiment and find out what works best for you. Be flexible. This includes trying different techniques and monitoring the results to see which technique is most helpful for which symptom(s) and under what circumstances.

- *Give yourself several weeks to practice a new symptom management technique* before you decide whether it is working for you. Remember that learning a new skill and gaining control of the situation take time.

- *Don't give up, even if you feel you are not accomplishing anything.* As is the case with exercise and other acquired skills, using your mind to manage your illness requires both practice and time before you notice the benefits. Be patient and keep on trying!

- *Self-management techniques should not have negative effects.* If you become frightened, angry, or depressed when using any one of these techniques, do not continue to use it. Try another technique instead.

and reflection are important parts of many people's self-management programs and remain the oldest of all symptom management techniques.

As we mentioned earlier in this book, symptoms, their causes, and the ways they interact to affect your daily life can become a vicious cycle. It is important to identify these symptoms and their causes in order to break the cycle and become a successful self-manager. On pages 3–5 and are some key principles to remember.

Suggested Reading

Borysenko, Joan. *Meditations for Relaxation and Stress Reduction.* Carlsbad, Calif.: Hay House, 1992.

Burns, David D. *Feeling Good: The New Mood Therapy.* New York: Avon Books, 1992.

Craze, Richard. *Teach Yourself Relaxation.* Chicago: Contemporary Publishing, 1998.

Davis, Martha, Eshelman, Elizabeth Robbins, and McKay, Matthew. *The Relaxation and Stress Reduction Workbook.* 2nd ed. Oakland, Calif.: New Harbinger Publications, 1988.

Kabat-Zinn, Jon. *Full Catastrophe Living: Using the Wisdom of Your Body to Face Stress, Pain and Illness.* New York: Delta, 1990.

Kabat-Zinn, Jon. *Wherever You Go, There You Are: Mindfulness Meditation in Everyday Life.* New York: Hyperion, 1995.

McKay, Matthew, and Fanning, Patrick. *The Daily Relaxer.* Oakland, Calif.: New Harbinger Publications, 1997.

McKay, Matthew, Fanning, Patrick, Honeychurch, Carole, and Sutker, Catherine. *The Self-Esteem Companion: Simple Exercises to Help Challenge Your Inner Critic and Celebrate Your Personal Strengths.* Oakland, Calif.: New Harbinger Publications, 1999.

Ornstein, Robert, and Sobel, David. *Healthy Pleasures.* Reading, Mass.: Addison-Wesley, 1989.

Rolek, Michiko J. *Mental Fitness: Complete Workouts for Body, Mind and Soul.* New York: Weatherhill, 1996.

Managing Exercise and Diet

10   Exercising for Fun and Fitness

Regular exercise and physical activity are vital to your physical and emotional health. They can also bring you fun and fitness. Having HIV/AIDS, however, can make it difficult to enjoy an active lifestyle. Some people may never have been really active, while others may have given up activities because of their condition. When you want to exercise but aren't sure what to do, physical and emotional limitations from HIV/AIDS can be powerful forces to overcome. Some people may even have been advised to avoid strenuous activity. Today, thanks to the knowledge gained from people with chronic health conditions who have worked with health professionals in exercise research, we know it is safe to advise exercise for fun and fitness.

Traditional medical care of chronic illness has been based mainly on helping people when their illness worsened, and has involved recommendations to decrease physical activity and increase medical therapy. Unfortunately, long periods of inactivity in anyone lead to weakness, stiffness, fatigue, poor appetite, constipation, high blood pressure, muscle loss, osteoporosis, and increased sensitivity to pain, anxiety, and depression. These same inactivity-related problems can be caused by the illness itself or by medications, so it can be difficult to tell whether it is the illness, medication, inactivity, or a combination of the three that is responsible for these problems. Although we cannot cure HIV/AIDS yet, we do know that exercise can cure inactivity.

Exercise can help you strengthen your immune system, maintain a healthy weight, improve your appetite, and control your blood sugar, fats, cholesterol, and blood pressure levels. In addition, exercise nourishes and strengthens your muscles and bones, helping to increase endurance and reduce fatigue and shortness of breath. Regular exercise is also an important part of reducing the risks of complications for those people who develop diabetes and high cholesterol from taking specific medications to control the progression of HIV disease.

Exercise reconditions your body, helping to restore function previously lost to disuse and illness. It will help you improve your health, feel better, and manage your illness better. Feeling more in control and less at the mercy of your illness is one of the biggest benefits of exercising.

In this chapter, you will learn how to improve your fitness and make wise exercise choices.*

Developing an Active Lifestyle

Okay, so you want to be more physically active. One way is to set aside a special time for a formal exercise program involving such planned activities as walking, jogging, swimming, tennis, dancing, or following an exercise videotape.

These kinds of formal programs are usually more visible and get more attention. But being more physical in everyday life can also pay off. Consider taking the stairs for a floor or two instead of waiting impatiently for a slow elevator. Park and walk the last few blocks to work or to the store instead of circling the parking lot looking for the perfect, up-close parking space. Play with the dog. Work in the garden. Just get up and walk around the house several times a day. These types of daily activities, often not viewed as "exercise," can add up to significant health benefits. Recent studies show that even small amounts of daily activity can raise fitness levels, improve strength, and improve your mood . . . and the activities can be pleasurable, enjoyable ones! One person commented that she *never* exercised. When asked why she went dancing several times a week, she replied, "Oh, that's not exercise, that's fun." The average day is filled with excellent opportunities to be more physical.

Developing an Exercise Program

Although you can get lots of exercise from the activities of daily life, a more formal exercise program can be helpful. Such a program usually involves setting aside a period of time, at least several times a week, to deliberately focus on increasing fitness.

---

*This advice is not intended to take the place of specific therapeutic recommendations from your doctor or physical therapist. If you've had an exercise plan prescribed for you that differs from the suggestions here, take this book to your doctor or physical therapist and ask what he or she thinks about this program.

A complete, balanced exercise program should help you improve these three aspects of fitness:

- *Flexibility.* This refers to the ability of the joints and muscles to move through a full, normal range of motion. Limited flexibility can cause pain, increase risk of injury, and make muscles less efficient. Flexibility tends to decrease with age and certain conditions, but you can increase or maximize your flexibility by doing gentle stretching exercises.

- *Strength.* Muscles need to be exercised to maintain their strength. With inactivity, they tend to weaken and shrink (atrophy). The weaker the muscles get, the less we feel like using them and the more inactive we tend to become, creating a vicious circle. Much of the disability and lack of mobility in people with HIV/AIDS is due to muscle weakness. This weakness can be reversed with a program that gradually increases exercise.

- *Endurance.* Our ability to sustain activity depends on certain vital capacities. The heart and lungs must work efficiently to distribute oxygen-rich blood to the muscles. The muscles must be conditioned to extract and utilize the oxygen.

    Aerobic (meaning "with oxygen") exercise conditions the heart, blood vessels, and muscles. This type of exercise uses the large muscles of your body in a rhythmical, continuous activity. The most effective activities involve your whole body: walking, swimming, dancing, mowing the lawn, and so on. Aerobic exercise improves cardiovascular fitness, lessens heart attack risk, and helps control weight. Aerobic exercise also promotes a sense of well-being—easing depression and anxiety, promoting restful sleep, and improving mood and energy levels.

A Good Fitness Program

A complete fitness program combines exercises to improve each of the three important aspects of fitness: flexibility, strength, and endurance. If you haven't exercised regularly in some time or have discomfort, stiffness, shortness of breath, or weakness that interferes with your daily activities, it is a good idea to talk with your health care providers before beginning your fitness program. Otherwise, start by choosing a number of flexibility and strengthening exercises that you are willing to do every day or every other day. Once you are able to exercise comfortably for at least ten minutes at a time, you are ready to add some endurance or aerobic activities.

Many people are uncertain about how to choose the right exercises and how to know what is best for them. The truth is that the best exercises are the ones that will help you do what you most want to do. Having a goal (something you want your exercise to help you achieve) is the most important ingredient of a successful fitness program. Once you have a goal in mind, it is much easier to choose exercises that make sense for you.

If you don't see how exercise can be helpful to you personally, it will be hard to get excited about adding yet another task to your day. The steps below may help you get started.

Choose your goal and make a plan

1. *Choose as a goal something that you want to do* but don't or can't do now because of some physical problem. For example, you might want to take a hiking trip with friends, paint your house, or prepare for a big celebration.

2. *Think about why you can't or don't do it or enjoy doing it now.* Maybe it is because you get tired before everybody else or you are too weak or short of breath to complete the activity.

3. *Decide what you can do to overcome the problem.* For example, you can gradually increase your endurance by walking a comfortable distance two or three times a week. Or you might practice deep breathing and strengthening exercises for your arms to help you manage your shortness of breath and upper body weakness.

4. *Design your exercise plan.* Choose no more than ten to twelve flexibility and strengthening exercises at first. Start by doing three to five repetitions of each, if you have not exercised for a while. As you improve, increase the number of repetitions and the number of exercises you do. If you want to improve endurance, first choose an aerobic activity you like (such as walking, swimming, bicycling, or dancing). Start off by doing this activity for short periods, or whatever you are comfortable doing now, and then build up gradually. Health and fitness take time to build, but every day you exercise makes you healthier and brings you closer to being fit. That's why it is important to keep it up.

Exercising for Endurance: How Much Is Enough?

One of the biggest problems with endurance (aerobic) exercise is that it is easy to overdo, even for people who don't have HIV/AIDS. Inexperienced and misinformed exercisers think they have to work very hard for exercise to do any good. Exhaustion, sore muscles, painful joints, and shortness of breath are the consequences of jumping in too hard and too fast. As a result, some people may put aside their exercise programs indefinitely, thinking that exercise is just not meant for them.

There is no magic formula for determining how much exercise you need. *The most important thing to remember is that some is better than none. Even a few minutes of exercise several times per week can be very beneficial.* If you start slowly and increase your efforts gradually, it is likely that you will maintain your exercise program as a lifelong habit. Generally, it is better to begin your conditioning program by underdoing rather than overdoing.

Several studies suggest that the *upper* limit of benefit is about 200 minutes of moderate-intensity aerobic exercise per week. Doing more than that doesn't gain you much (and it increases your risk of injury). On the other hand, doing 100 minutes of exercise per week gets you about 90 percent of the gain, whereas 60 minutes of aerobic exercise per week yields about 75 percent of the gain. Sixty minutes is just 15 minutes of mild aerobic exercise four times a week!

Following are some general guidelines for the frequency, duration, and intensity of aerobic exercise.

- *Frequency.* Try to exercise three or four times a week. Taking every other day off gives your body a chance to rest and recover. We recommend that you rest at least one day per week.

- *Duration.* Start with just a few minutes, and then gradually increase the duration of your aerobic activity to about 30 minutes a session. You can safely increase the time by alternating intervals of brisk exercise with intervals of rest or easy exercise. For example, after 3 to 5 minutes of brisk walking, do 1 to 2 minutes of easy strolling and then another 3 to 5 minutes of brisk walking. Eventually, you can build up to 30 minutes of activity. Then gradually eliminate rest intervals until you can maintain 20 to 30 minutes of brisk exercise. If 30 minutes seems too long, consider two sessions of 10 to 15 minutes each; either way appears to improve fitness levels significantly.

- *Intensity.* Safe and effective endurance exercise should be done at no more than *moderate intensity.* High-intensity exercise increases the risk of injury and causes discomfort, so not many people stick with it. Exercise intensity is measured by how hard you work. For a trained runner, completing a mile in 12 minutes is probably low-intensity exercise. For a person who hasn't exercised in a long time, a brisk 10-minute walk may be of moderate to high intensity. For others with severe physical limitations, 1 minute may be of moderate intensity.

Remember, these are just rough guidelines on frequency, duration, and intensity, not a rigid prescription. Listen to your own body. Sometimes you need to tell yourself (and maybe others) that enough is enough. More exercise is not necessarily better, especially if it gives you pain or discomfort. As *Walking* magazine says, "Go for the smiles, not the miles."

You can determine your own individual intensity guidelines through several intensity-monitoring techniques: the talk test, perceived exertion, and heart rate.

Talk Test

Talk to another person or yourself, sing, or recite poems out loud while you exercise. Moderate-intensity exercise allows you to speak comfortably. If you can't carry on a conversation or sing because you are breathing too hard or are short of breath, you're working too hard. Slow down. The talk test is an easy way to regulate exercise intensity.

If you have breathing problems, the talk test might not work for you. If that is the case, try the perceived exertion test.

Perceived Exertion

Another way to monitor intensity is to rate how hard you're working on a scale of 0 to 10. Zero, at the low end of the scale, is lying down, doing no work at all. Ten is equivalent to working as hard as possible—very hard work that you couldn't do longer than a few seconds. Of course, you never want to exercise that hard. A good level for your aerobic exercise routine is between 3 and 6 on this scale. At this level, you'll usually perspire and breathe faster and more deeply than usual, and your heart will beat faster than normal, but you should not be feeling pain.

Heart Rate

Monitoring your heart rate while exercising is another way to measure exercise intensity. The faster the heart beats, the harder you're working. (Your heart also beats fast when you are frightened or nervous, but here we're talking about how your heart responds to physical activity.) Endurance exercise at moderate intensity raises your heart rate into a range between 60 and 80 percent of your safe maximum heart rate. The safe maximum heart rate declines with age, so your safe exercise heart rate gets lower as you get older. You can follow the general guidelines of the following Exercise Heart Rate chart, or you can calculate your individual exercise heart rate. Either way, you need to know how to take your pulse.

Take your pulse by placing the tips of your middle three fingers at your wrist below the base of your thumb. Feel around in that spot until you feel the pulsations of blood pumping with each heartbeat. Count how many beats you feel in 15 seconds. Multiply this number by 4 to find out how fast your heart is beating in 1 minute. Start by taking your pulse whenever you think of it, and you'll soon learn the difference between your resting and exercise heart rates.

How to calculate your own ideal exercise heart rate range

1. Subtract your age from 220:
   Example: 220 – 40 = 180   *You:* 220 – _____ = _____

Exercise Heart Rate	
Age Range	*Exercise Pulse (beats per 15 seconds)*
20–30	29–39
30–40	28–37
40–50	26–35
50–60	25–33
60–70	23–31
70–80	22–29
80+	16–24

2. To find the *lower end* of your
    exercise heart rate range, multiply
    your answer in step 1 by 0.6.

    Example: 180 × 0.6 = 108   You: _____ × 0.6 = _____

3. To find the *upper end* of your
    exercise heart rate range, *which
    you should not exceed,* multiply
    your answer in step 1 by 0.8.

    Example: 180 × 0.8 = 144   You: _____ × 0.8 = _____

The exercise heart rate range in our example is from 108 to 144 beats per minute. What is yours?

Most people count their pulse for 15 seconds, not a whole minute. To find your 15-second pulse, divide both numbers by 4. The person in our example should be able to count between 24 and 32 beats in 15 seconds while exercising.

The most important reason to know your ideal exercise heart rate range is so that you can learn not to exercise too vigorously. After you've done your warm-up and 5 minutes of endurance exercise, take your pulse. If it's *higher than the upper rate, don't panic.* Slow down a bit. Don't work so hard.

At first, some people have trouble keeping their heart rate within the ideal exercise heart rate range. Don't worry about that. Keep exercising at the level with which you're most comfortable. As you get more experienced and stronger, you will gradually be able to do more vigorous exercise while keeping your heart rate within your "goal" range. But don't let the target heart rate monitoring become a burden. Recent studies have shown that even low-intensity exercise can provide significant health benefits. So use the ideal heart rate range as a rough guide, but don't worry if you can't reach the lower end of that range. The important thing is to keep exercising!

If you are taking medicine that regulates your heart rate, have trouble feeling your pulse, or think that keeping track of your heart rate is a bother, use one of the other methods to monitor your exercise intensity.

When to Warm Up and Cool Down

If you are going to exercise at an intensity that causes you to breathe harder or your heart to beat faster, it is important to warm up first. A warm-up means that you do at least 5 minutes of a low-intensity activity to allow your heart, lungs, and circulation to gradually increase their work. If you are going for a brisk walk, warm up with five minutes of slow walking first. If you are riding a stationary bike, warm up with 5 minutes of no resistance at no more than 60 rpm. In an aerobic exercise class, you will warm up with a gentle routine before moving on to more vigorous activity. Warming up reduces the risk of injury, soreness, and irregular heartbeat.

A cooldown period is also important after you have exercised at an intensity that has made you breathe harder, feel warm or perspire, or caused your heart to beat faster. Repeating the 5-minute warm-up activity or taking a slow walk helps your muscles to gradually relax, and your heart and breathing to slow down. Gentle flexibility and strengthening exercises during the cooldown can help increase your range of motion and reduce muscle soreness and stiffness.

You might enjoy a routine of flexibility and strengthening exercises that you can use as part of your warm-up and cooldown periods. If you do so, arrange the exercises so that they flow together and you don't have to get up and down too much. Also, try exercising to gentle, rhythmic music to make it more enjoyable. Following are some tips on how to do these exercises properly.

The *FIT* Formula

The results of your aerobic exercise program depend on how often you exercise (*F* = frequency), how hard you work (*I* = intensity), and how long you exercise each day (*T* = time). In much the same way that a doctor prescribes medicine to produce a certain effect, you can select your own dosage of exercise to get the results you want. Your exercise dosage comes from how you combine the frequency, intensity, and time of your exercise. Within the limits of safety and common sense, the bigger the dosage, the greater the effect.

- *Frequency:* Three to five days a week. Three days a week is the starting minimum. As you gain endurance and strength, you can do aerobic exercise and activities more often. If you exercise more vigorously, three days is enough. If your aerobic exercise is a comfortably paced walk, you can build up to five or even seven days a week.

- *Intensity:* No more than moderate. This means being able to carry on a conversation while you exercise, a perceived exertion level of no more than 6, or an exercise heart rate of no more than 75 percent of your age-predicted maximum heart rate.

- *Time:* At least 30 minutes of mild to moderate physical activity in a day. The activity may be divided into 10-minute periods. To improve cardiovascular fitness, you may need to exercise a bit longer each time.

The U. S. Surgeon General's Report on Physical Activity recommends that *adults accumulate 30 minutes of moderate physical activity on most days of the week.* This is the goal, but it may not be the starting point for every person. If you begin exercising just 2 minutes at a time, however, you are likely to be able to reach 10 minutes of exercise or physical activity, three times a day. You are also likely to achieve your personal exercise goal and other health benefits.

What Are Your Exercise Barriers?

Fitness makes sense. Yet when faced with the prospect of actually becoming more physically active, most people can come up with scores of excuses, concerns, and worries. These barriers can prevent us from even taking the first step. Following are some common barriers and possible solutions.

I don't have enough time.

Everyone has the same amount of time; we just choose to use it differently. It's a matter of priorities. Some find a lot of time for television, but nothing to spare for fitness. It doesn't really take a lot of time. Even five minutes a day is a good start, and much better than no physical activity. You may be able to combine activities, such as watching television while pedaling a stationary bicycle, or arranging "walking meetings" to discuss business or family matters.

I'm too tired.

When you're out of shape, you feel listless and tend to tire easily. Then you don't exercise because you're tired, and this becomes a vicious cycle. You have to break out of the being-tired cycle. Regular physical activity increases your stamina and gives you more energy to do the things you like. As you get back into shape, you will recognize the difference between feeling listless or out of shape and feeling physically tired.

Helpful Tips for Doing Flexibility and Strengthening Exercises

- *Move slowly and gently.* Do not bounce or jerk. Those movements actually tighten and shorten muscles.
- To loosen tight muscles and limber up stiff joints, *stretch just until you feel tension,* hold for 5 to 10 seconds, and then relax.
- *Don't push your body until it hurts.* Stretching should feel good, not painful.
- *Start with no more than five repetitions of any exercise.* Take at least two weeks to increase to ten.
- Always do the *same number* of exercises for your left side as for your right.
- *Breathe naturally.* Do not hold your breath. Count out loud to make sure you are breathing easily.
- If you feel increased symptoms that last more than *2 hours* after exercising, next time do fewer repetitions, or eliminate the exercise that seems to be causing the symptoms. *Don't quit exercising.*
- *All exercises can be adapted to individual needs.* If you are limited by muscle weakness or joint tightness, go ahead and do the exercise as completely as you can. The benefit of doing an exercise comes from moving toward a certain position, not from being able to complete the movement perfectly the first time. In some cases you may find that after a while you can complete the movement. Other times you will continue to perform your own version.

I'm too sick.

It may be true that you are too sick for a vigorous or strenuous exercise program, but you can usually find some ways to be more active. Remember, you can exercise one minute at a time, several times a day. The enhanced physical fitness you will gain can help you better cope with your illness and prevent further problems.

I get enough exercise.

This may be true, but for most people, their jobs and daily activities do not provide enough sustained exercise to keep them fully fit and energetic.

Exercise is boring.

You can make it more interesting and fun. Exercise with other people. Entertain yourself with a headset and musical tapes, or listen to the radio. Vary your activities and your walking routes.

Exercise is painful.

The old saying "No pain, no gain" is simply wrong and out of date. Recent evidence shows that significant health benefits come from gentle, low-intensity, enjoyable physical activity. You may sweat or feel a bit short of breath, but if you feel more pain than before you started, something is probably wrong. More than likely you are either exercising improperly or you're overdoing it. Talk with your physician. You may simply need to be less vigorous or change the type of exercise that you're doing.

I'm too embarrassed.

For some, the thought of donning a skintight designer exercise outfit and trotting around in public is delightful, but for others it is downright distressing. Fortunately, the options for physical activity range from exercise in the privacy of your own home to group social activities. You should be able to find something that suits you.

It's too cold, it's too hot, it's too dark. . . .

If you are flexible and vary your type of exercise, you can generally work around the changes in weather that make certain types of exercise more difficult. Consider indoor activities such as stationary bicycling or working out at the gym.

I'm afraid I won't be able to do it right or be successful.
I'm afraid I'll fail.

Many people don't start a new project because they are afraid they will fail or not be able to finish it successfully. If you feel this way about starting an exercise program, remember two things. First, whatever activities you are able to do—no matter how short or "easy"—will be much better for you than doing nothing. Be proud of what you *have* done, not guilty about what you *haven't* done. Second, new projects often seem overwhelming—until you get started and learn to enjoy each day's adventures and successes.

Perhaps you have come up with some other barriers. The human mind is incredibly creative. But you can turn that creativity to your advantage by using it to come up with even better ways to refute the excuses and develop positive attitudes about exercise and fitness. If you get stuck, ask others for suggestions, or try some of the self-talk suggestions in Chapter 9.

Preparing to Exercise

Figuring out how to make the commitment of time and energy toward regular exercise is a challenge for everyone. If you have HIV/AIDS and are following complicated medication schedules, you have even more challenges. You may need to take precautions and find a safe, comfortable program. Even with AIDS, most people can do some kind of aerobic exercise.

If your illness is not stable, if you have been inactive for more than six months, or if you have questions about starting an aerobic exercise program, it is best to check with your health care provider first. Take this book with you when you discuss your exercise ideas, or prepare a list of your specific questions.

You should understand how to adapt your exercise to changes in your condition. For example, do not "exercise through" potentially serious symptoms, such as chest pain, shortness of breath, or excessive fatigue. Notify your physician of any significant worsening of your usual symptoms or appearance of new symptoms. Go back to exercising only after getting the physician's clearance to do so. Also, don't exercise when you are experiencing flu symptoms, an upset stomach, diarrhea, or another acute illness.

Learning how much to push yourself while exercising without doing "too much" is especially important. We hope that this chapter will help you to meet these challenges and enjoy the benefits of physical fitness. Start by identifying your individual needs and limits. If possible, talk with your doctor and other health professionals. Get their ideas about special exercise needs and precautions. Learn to be aware of your body, and plan activities accordingly. Respect your body. If you feel acutely ill, don't exercise. If you can't comfortably complete your warm-up period of flexibility and strengthening exercises, then don't try to do more vigorous conditioning exercises. Your personal exercise program should be based on *your* current level of health and fitness, *your* goals and desires, *your* abilities and special needs, and *your* likes and dislikes. Deciding to improve your fitness and feeling the satisfaction of success have nothing to do with competition or comparing yourself with others.

Opportunities in Your Community

Most people who exercise regularly do so with at least one other person. Two or more people can keep each other motivated, and a whole class can build a feeling of camaraderie. On the other hand, exercising alone gives you the most freedom. You may feel that there are no classes that would work for you, or no buddy with whom you can exercise. If so, start your own program; as you progress, you may find that these feelings change.

Many communities now offer a variety of exercise classes, including special programs for people with health problems, adaptive exercises, tai chi, yoga, fitness trails, and others. Check with the local Y, community centers, parks and recreation programs, adult education, and community colleges. There is a great deal of variation in the content of these programs, as well as in the professional experience of the exercise staff. By and large, the classes are inexpensive, and those in charge of planning are responsive to people's needs.

Health and fitness clubs usually offer aerobic studios, weight training, cardiovascular equipment, and sometimes a heated pool. For all these services they charge membership fees, which can be high. But some clubs have discounts for people with chronic illness. Ask about low-impact and beginners' exercise classes, both in the aerobic studio and in the pool.* Gyms that emphasize weight lifting generally don't have the programs or personnel to help you with a flexible, overall fitness program.

In choosing an exercise class or a health and fitness club, look for the following qualities:

- Classes designed for *moderate- and low-intensity* exercise. You should be able to observe classes and participate in at least one class before signing up and paying.

- Instructors with *qualifications and experience.* Knowledgeable instructors are more likely to understand special needs and be willing and able to work with you.

- Membership policies that allow you to pay for only a session of classes, or let you "freeze" membership at times when you can't

---

*You may be wondering whether it's safe for others if you use a public pool or exercise/fitness equipment. Are you putting other people at risk for catching HIV from you? Let's be clear here, because we don't want you avoiding exercise out of concern for others: *It is not dangerous for you to use public pools or exercise equipment or to play group sports.* No one has ever caught HIV from any kind of group sport or exercise. So just use common sense. If you're bleeding, stop your exercise and clean up after yourself. All people should do the same, whether they have HIV or not.

participate. Some fitness facilities offer *different rates* depending on how many services you use.

- Facilities that are *easy to get to, park near, and enter.* Dressing rooms and exercise sites should be accessible and safe, with professional staff on site.

- A pool that allows *"free swim"* times when the water isn't crowded. Also, find out the policy about children in the pool; small children playing and making noise may not be compatible with your program.

- Staff and other members whom you *feel comfortable* being around.

One last note: There are many excellent videotapes for home use. They vary in intensity from very gentle chair exercises to more strenuous aerobic exercise. Ask your doctor, physical therapist, or voluntary agency for suggestions, or review the tapes yourself.

Putting Your Program Together

The best way to enjoy and stick with your exercise program is to *suit yourself!* Choose what you want to do, a place where you feel comfortable, and an exercise time that fits your schedule.

Pick two or three activities you think you would enjoy and that won't put undue stress on your body. Choose activities that can be easily worked into your daily routine. If an activity is new to you, try it out before going to the expense of buying equipment or joining a health club. By practicing more than one exercise, you can keep active while adapting to vacations, seasons, and changing problems with your illness. Variety also helps keep you from getting bored.

Having fun and enjoying yourself are benefits of exercise that often go unmentioned. Too often we think of exercise as serious business. However, most people who stick with a program do so because they enjoy it. *They think of their exercise as recreation rather than as a chore.* Start off with success in mind. Allow yourself time to get used to new experiences, and you'll probably find that you look forward to exercise.

Some well-meaning health professionals can make it hard for a person with health problems to stick to an exercise program. You may have been told simply to "exercise more" on your own. The how and when of that exercise plan, in fact, may have been left entirely up to you. No wonder so many people never start or give up so quickly! Not many of us would make a commitment to do something we don't fully understand. Experience, practice, and success help us establish a habit. Follow the self-management steps described in Chapter 2 to make beginning your program easier.

- *Keep your exercise goal in mind.*
- *Choose exercises you want to do.* Combine activities that move you toward your goal and are recommended by your health care providers.
- *Choose the time and place to exercise.* Tell your partner, family, and friends your plan.
- *Make an action plan for yourself.* Decide how long you'll stick with these particular exercises. Six to eight weeks is a reasonable time commitment for a new program.
- *Try keeping an exercise diary* or calendar, leaving space to write down your exercises, how long you do them, your heart rate or perceived exertion score, and your feelings before and after exercise. Put your diary where you can see it, and fill it out every day.
- *Do some self-tests to keep track of your progress.* Distance and time self-tests appear on page 155. Record the date and results. You may also use your exercise diary for this purpose.
- *Start your program.* Remember to begin gradually and proceed slowly, especially if you haven't exercised in a while.
- *Repeat the self-tests* at regular intervals, record the results, and check the changes.
- *Revise your program.* At the end of six to eight weeks, decide what you liked, what worked, and what made exercising difficult. Modify your program and make another action plan for the next few weeks. You may decide to change some exercises, the place or time that you exercise, or your exercise partners.
- *Reward yourself for a job well done.* Many people who start an exercise program find that the rewards come with improved fitness and endurance. Being able to enjoy outings, a refreshing walk, or trips to a store, the library, a concert, or a museum are great rewards to look forward to.

Self-Tests for Endurance and Aerobic Fitness

For some people, just the feelings of increased endurance and well-being are enough to indicate progress. Others may find it helpful to demonstrate that their exercise program is making a measurable difference. You may wish to try one or both of the following endurance and aerobic fitness tests before you start

Distance Self-Test

- Find a place to walk or bicycle where you can measure distance. A running track works well. On a street you can measure distance with a car. A stationary bicycle with an odometer provides the equivalent measurement. If you plan on swimming, you can count pool lengths.

- After a warm-up, note your starting point and either bicycle, swim, or walk as briskly as you *comfortably* can for 5 minutes. Try to move at a steady pace for the full time. At the end of 5 minutes, mark your spot and immediately take your pulse and rate your perceived exertion from 0 to 10. Continue at a slow pace for 3 to 5 more minutes to cool down. Measure and record the distance, your heart rate, and your perceived exertion.

- Repeat the test after several weeks of exercise. There may be a change in as little as 4 weeks. However, it often takes 8 to 12 weeks to see improvement.

Goal: To cover more distance *or* to lower your heart rate *or* to lower your perceived exertion.

Time Self-Test

- Measure a given distance to walk, bike, or swim. Estimate how far you think you can go in 1 to 5 minutes. You can pick a number of blocks, actual distance, or lengths in a pool.

- Spend 3 to 5 minutes warming up. Start timing and start moving steadily, briskly, and comfortably. At the finish, record how long it took you to cover your course, your heart rate, and your perceived exertion.

- Repeat after several weeks of exercise. You may see changes in as soon as 4 weeks. However, it often takes 8 to 12 weeks for a noticeable improvement.

Goal: To complete the course in less time *or* at a lower heart rate *or* at a lower perceived exertion.

your exercise program. Not everyone will be able to do both tests, so pick the one that works best for you. Record your results in your exercise diary. After four weeks of exercise, do the test again and check your improvement. Measure your progress again after four more weeks.

Maintaining Your Commitment to Exercise

If you haven't exercised recently, you'll undoubtedly experience some new feelings and discomfort in the early days. Most of these new feelings are normal and expected, but a few might mean you should change what you're doing. See "Advice for Exercise Problems" on page 157 if you're concerned. But remember, it's normal to feel muscle tension and tenderness around joints and to be a little more tired in the evenings. *Muscle or joint pain that lasts more than two hours after the exercise, or feeling tired into the next day, means that you probably did too much too fast. Don't stop;* just exercise less vigorously or for a shorter amount of time the next day.

When you do aerobic exercise, it's natural to feel your heart beat faster, your breathing speed up, and your body get warmer. However, irregular or very rapid heartbeats, excessive shortness of breath, or dizziness are not what you want. If this happens to you, stop exercising and discontinue your program until you check with your doctor.

If you have symptoms such as fatigue, shortness of breath, or physical discomfort, it can be difficult at first to figure out whether these are caused by the illness, medication, exercise, or some combination of these. Talking to someone else with HIV/AIDS about his or her experience in starting an exercise program may help. Once you are able to sort out some of these sensations, you'll be able to exercise with confidence.

Expect setbacks. During the first year of an exercise program, people average two to three interruptions in their exercise schedule, often because of minor injuries or illnesses unrelated to their exercise. You may find yourself sidelined or derailed temporarily. Don't be discouraged. Try a different activity or simply rest. When you are feeling better, resume your program, but begin at a lower, more gentle level. As a rule of thumb, it will take you the same amount of time to get back into shape as you were out. For instance, if you missed three weeks, it may take at least three weeks to get back to your previous level. Go slowly. Be kind to yourself. You're in this for the long haul.

Think of your head as the coach and your body as the team. For success, all parts of your team need attention. Be a good coach. *Encourage and praise yourself.* Design "plays" you feel your team can execute successfully. Choose places that are safe and hospitable. A good coach knows his or her team, sets good goals, and helps the team succeed. A good coach is loyal. A good coach does not belittle, nag, or make anyone feel guilty. Be a good coach to your team.

Besides a good coach, everyone needs an enthusiastic cheerleader or two. Of course, you can be your own cheerleader, but being both coach and cheerleader is a lot to do. A successful exerciser usually has at least one *family member or close friend who actively supports* his or her exercise habit. Your cheerleader can exercise with you, help you get chores done, praise your accomplishments, or just consider your exercise time when making plans. Sometimes cheerleaders pop up by themselves, but don't be bashful about asking for a hand.

Advice for Exercise Problems

Problem	Advice
Irregular or very rapid heartbeat	Stop exercising. Check your pulse. Are the beats regular or irregular? How fast is your heartbeat? Make a note of this information, and discuss it with your doctor before exercising again.
Pain, tightness, or pressure in your chest, jaw, arms, neck, or back	Stop exercising and sit or lie down. If the pain, tightness, or pressure lasts more than 15 minutes, see a doctor right away. Check with your doctor about these symptoms before exercising again.
Unusual, extreme shortness of breath, persisting 10 minutes after you exercise	Notify your doctor and get clearance before exercising again.
Lightheadedness, dizziness, fainting, cold sweat, or confusion	Lie down with your feet up, or sit down and put your head between your legs. If it happens more than once, check with your doctor before exercising again.
Excessive tiredness after exercise, especially if you're still tired 24 hours after you exercise	Don't exercise so vigorously next time. If the excessive tiredness persists, check with your doctor.

With exercise experience you develop a sense of control in your life. You learn how to *alternate your activities to fit your day-to-day needs.* You know when to do less and when to do more. You know that a change in symptoms or a period of inactivity is usually only temporary and doesn't have to be devastating. You know you have the tools to get back on track again.

Give your exercise plan a chance to succeed. Set reasonable goals and enjoy your success. Stay motivated. When it comes to your personal fitness program, sticking with it and doing it your way makes you a definite winner.

Resources

- Adult education
- Community colleges
- Health and fitness clubs

- Hospitals, health care organizations
- Parks and recreation programs
- YMCA, YWCA

Suggested Reading

Cooper, Kenneth H. *The Aerobics Program for Total Well-Being: Exercise, Diet, Emotional Balance.* New York: Bantam Doubleday, 1985.

Green, Tamara. *Exercise Is Fun! Good Health Guidelines.* Milwaukee: Gareth Stevens, 1998.

Nelson, Miriam E. *Strong Women Stay Young.* New York: Bantam Books, 1998.

Stewart, Gordon W. *Active Living: The Miracle of Medicine for a Long and Healthy Life.* Champaign, Ill.: Human Kinetics, 1995.

Torkelson, Charlene. *Get Fit While You Sit: Easy Workout from Your Chair.* Berkeley: Hunter House, 1999.

Vedral, Joyce L. *Bone Building and Body Shaping Workout.* New York: Simon & Schuster, 1998.

Weddington, Michael. *Aerobic Sports Log: A Revolutionary Graphical Log Book for the Health Conscious Individual.* Griffin Bay Book Store, 1997.

White, Martha. *Water Exercise: 78 Safe and Effective Exercises for Fitness and Therapy.* Champaign, Ill.: Human Kinetics, 1995.

11   Healthy Eating

Eating healthy foods is important at any time, but even more so when you are HIV positive. A nutritionally balanced eating plan gives you more energy and strength to carry out your daily activities and enjoy life as much as possible. It also helps your body's immune system to fight off infections and can even prevent other health problems. Although there is currently no cure for HIV disease, we do know that healthy eating helps to slow the disease process, prevent weight loss, and control some of the unpleasant side effects of medications, thereby contributing to the quality of your life.

In this chapter we offer some guidelines for you to consider in developing an eating plan. We also discuss ways to manage some of the common eating problems associated with HIV disease and medication side effects. In Chapter 12, we provide important tips on food safety and preparation. Just as with the other self-management techniques discussed in this book, putting these suggestions into practice can help you feel more in control of your condition and your life.

What Is Healthy Eating?

Figuring out what foods to eat is one of the most common concerns of people with HIV disease, especially since disease symptoms or medications often interfere with the ability or desire to eat. Unfortunately, there is no one answer, but there is a general guideline to follow: eat a variety of healthy foods in the appropriate amounts regularly throughout the day. The specific amounts of these foods and how many times a day to eat, however, will vary depending on your specific health condition, nutritional needs, and eating problems. To help you establish your own eating plan, we ask you to keep the following basic principles of healthy eating in mind.

Principles of healthy eating

- Eat a variety of foods from each of the food groups every day.
- Eat small, frequent meals or have snacks at least four times per day.
- Drink plenty of fluids each day (at least eight full glasses).
- Increase the amount of protein and calories you eat (if your weight is below normal, if you are not eating enough, or if you have chronic diarrhea).
- Take a multivitamin/mineral supplement every day.
- Avoid chemical stimulants, such as:
  - caffeine (coffee, some dark teas, regular sodas)
  - alcoholic drinks (beer, wine, and liquor)
  - recreational drugs (cigarettes, cigars, cocaine, marijuana, "speed," etc.)

Eating a variety of foods from the different food groups every day helps you get all the nutrients your body needs to function well. These nutrients include protein, carbohydrates, fats, vitamins, minerals, and water. Each nutrient plays an important role in your body. Unfortunately, no one food contains them all; therefore, we must eat a variety of foods from different groups. The nutrients and the foods in which they are commonly found are listed in the table on page 162.

Eating small, frequent meals or snacks throughout the day provides you with the energy needed to maintain your bodily functions and muscle weight. It also helps your body absorb and use medications, and it lessens some of the medications' side effects. It is especially important to eat small, frequent meals if you have been losing weight—particularly muscle mass and protein. Such weight loss may occur when you have little or no appetite and are not eating enough. It might also be the result of your body fighting off an infection or other illness; this causes your metabolism to increase and use more energy. In addition, you may experience loss of weight and nutrients as a result of chronic diarrhea. If you are losing weight for one of these reasons, you may need to modify your eating plan to include more protein and/or calories as well as vitamins and minerals. Some general tips for doing this are listed on page 173. You might also consider talking with your doctor or nutritionist about other ways to adjust your eating plan if you continue to have problems.

Drinking plenty of fluids every day is vital, especially if you are taking medications. Your body needs water in order to function normally, to use nutrients and medications efficiently, and to eliminate waste and toxins. Because the body uses water to help flush out medications, you must take in more fluid to prevent dehydration. We recommend that you drink at least eight full glasses of water and other liquids each day. If you are taking many medications, drink more liquid. If you are having difficulty maintaining your weight or eating food, try drinking high-calorie fluids (juices, nectars, Gatorade) or high-protein drinks (milk, milk shakes, fortified milk, soy milk, Ensure Plus, Nutren 2.0, Nutrament, Resource Plus, Sustacal) in place of or in addition to water. Try to avoid drinks that contain caffeine (coffee, some dark teas, and some sodas) or alcohol. Not only are these types of drinks low in nutrients, but they also dehydrate you.

Because some germs can be spread through tap water, it is better to drink bottled water. This can be distilled water, spring water filtered to 2 microns, or carbonated soda water. If you want to use tap water to drink or to make ice cubes or juices, boil the water for at least five minutes and let it cool. If you drink bottled juices, choose those that are pasteurized to avoid bacteria that can make you sick, especially when your immune system is suppressed.

You may benefit from *taking daily multivitamin and mineral supplements*. Deficiencies in vitamins A, B6, and C and in minerals such as zinc, selenium, iron, and copper can worsen the immune suppression caused by not eating enough protein and calories.

If you are HIV positive and asymptomatic, we recommend that you take a multivitamin and mineral supplement that provides 100 percent of the U.S. recommended dietary allowance (RDA) daily. The RDA is a standard level set by the government that has been determined to prevent deficiencies and maintain health.

If you are symptomatic, we recommend that you take two supplement pills (200 percent of the RDA) daily with your meals. Research has shown that as the HIV disease progresses, you can become deficient in other vitamins or minerals (such as vitamin B12 and folate). To determine whether or not you need higher doses of certain vitamins and minerals, ask your doctor to check your blood levels when you have your regular blood work done.

Many people choose to take therapeutic doses of these and other vitamins and minerals (such as beta-carotene, vitamin E, and vitamin C) to prevent deficiencies and enhance the body's immune function. If you decide to begin therapeutic doses of vitamins and minerals, discuss this with your doctor. High doses or overdoses of certain vitamins and minerals (particularly vitamins A, D, and B6, and zinc, selenium, iron, and copper) can cause serious side effects, such as nausea, diarrhea, and loss of appetite; they can even damage your liver and kidneys. Taking more than the recommended doses of vitamins and minerals is considered a type of drug therapy, and therefore should be supervised by your physician.

Essential Nutrients, Their Functions, and Food Sources

Nutrient	Functions	Food Sources
Proteins	• Build and repair muscle and organ tissues • Build enzymes and hormones • Fight off infection • Maintain the body's immune system • Provide energy	Animal sources include red meat, fish, poultry, organ meats, eggs, and dairy products. These provide complete proteins. Vegetable sources include legumes (beans and peas), grains, cereals, nuts, seeds, tofu, and other soy products. These are incomplete proteins but when eaten together in the right combinations make complete proteins. They provide fiber and contain no saturated fat.
Carbohydrates	• Provide the major source of energy for the body's metabolism and muscles • Help build and maintain muscles	Starches or complex carbohydrates include grains, rice, pasta, breads, cereals, legumes (peas and beans), and vegetables. Sugars or simple carbohydrates include fruits and some dairy products. Other sources of simple sugars include processed foods made with table sugar, honey, syrups, and jellies (cakes, candies, etc.). These provide extra calories but have little or no nutritional value.
Fats	• Provide extra energy to burn, and build body fat • Help build, strengthen, and repair tissues • If eaten in excess, lead to weight gain	Meat, whole-milk dairy products, nuts, peanuts, seeds, oils, salad dressings, and processed products such as cakes and candies Eat only moderate amounts of fats, especially saturated fats, which come from the animal sources listed above.

	(continued)	
Nutrient	*Functions*	*Food Sources*
Vitamins and minerals	• Help build strong bones and muscles • Are involved in specific reactions in your body to ensure that it functions properly	These are found in varying amounts in all the different food groups, and interact with the other nutrients in the body. Multivitamin and mineral supplements may be necessary if you are HIV positive, because your body may need more nutrients than food provides. This is especially true if you have a poor appetite or skip meals, are fighting off infections, or have chronic diarrhea.
Water	• Helps dissolve nutrients and carries them to all parts of the body to be used as energy • Flushes out the body's toxins and waste products • Prevents dehydration and lessens some medication side effects (e.g., dry mouth and constipation)	All foods contain water. Major sources include broth, ice pops, and gelatin. Avoid drinks with caffeine or alcohol; these increase water loss by stimulating urination and causing diarrhea.

Good brands of over-the-counter (nonprescription) supplements include Centrum and Theragran-M. You may also ask your doctor to write a prescription for a multivitamin and mineral supplement that is covered by Medicaid or your state's AIDS Drug Assistance Program (ADAP). If you are considering prescription rather than over-the-counter supplements and are planning to take doses higher than the recommended daily allowances, find out if this is covered by your insurance. (As of this writing, such higher doses are not covered, which means you must pay the costs yourself.)

Recommended Daily Servings of Different Food Groups

Food Group	Recommended Servings per Day	Examples of Servings
Protein	3	2–3 ounces of cooked meat, fish, or poultry 2 cooked eggs 4 tablespoons of peanut butter (or other nut butter) 1 cup of cooked dried beans or peas ½ cup of nuts or seeds 5–6 ounces of tofu
Dairy	3	1 cup milk 1 cup yogurt 1 cup ice cream or frozen yogurt ½ cup cottage cheese 1–2 ounces of cheese
Starches: breads, cereal, rice, pasta	8–11	1 slice of bread ½ of an English muffin, bagel, or bun 1 cup of flake-type cereal ½ cup of cooked cereal ½ cup of cooked pasta or rice 2 flour or corn tortillas 6 saltine-type crackers 3 squares of graham crackers
Vegetables	4 or more	1 cup of raw leafy vegetables (washed thoroughly) ½ cup of other vegetables, cooked or chopped raw (washed thoroughly) ¾ cup of vegetable juice
Fruits	3	1 medium-sized apple, banana, orange or other whole fruit (washed well or peeled) ½ cup of chopped, cooked, or canned fruit ¾ cup of fruit juice ¼ cup of dried fruit

	(continued)	
Food Group	*Recommended Servings per Day*	*Examples of Servings*
Fats and sweets	Moderate use only, unless you need to take in more calories	Margarine, salad dressings, sour cream, and mayonnaise Sugar, jelly, jam, honey, and syrup

Making a Healthy Eating Plan

Designing and following a healthy eating plan can be difficult. After all, it involves changing eating habits that you have had for many years. Changing what you eat, how you prepare your food, and how often you eat are not easy things to do, especially if you try to do them all at once. Therefore, to be successful, it is helpful to break your goal into smaller, more manageable steps. This is the essence of being a self-manager.

Step 1: Identify Why You Want to Change Your Eating Plan

This will help motivate you to get started and to stick with the changes you want or need to make. The reasons for changing eating habits differ for each individual. The most obvious reason, if you have HIV disease, is to maintain your physical health, but you may also have psychological or emotional reasons for wanting to change. Determine for yourself why you want to make changes. For example, you may want to:

- lessen disease symptoms or medication side effects, such as nausea, diarrhea, pain, or fatigue
- have more energy for the things you want to do
- feel better about yourself
- strengthen your resistance to infections and other common illnesses
- change the way others perceive you
- feel more in control of your disease and your life

If you have other reasons, jot them down below. You may want to review these periodically to remind yourself of their importance and to help motivate you when you are tempted to give up.

_____

_____

_____

Step 2: Look at What You Eat Now and What You Want or Need to Change

Start by keeping track of what you are currently eating. Look at yesterday's meals. Use the food diary on page 167 to list all the foods you ate (including snacks) and the amount or portion size of each. (If you don't want to use this diary, make your own.) If you ate a mixed dish (e.g., pasta with sauce, casserole, or soup), try to estimate how much of each food group was in your serving of that dish. Use the portion sizes listed on pages 164–165 to determine the number of servings you had of each food group for the day. Write the total number of servings you had for the day and compare this to the recommended minimum number of servings for that food group.

You may want to keep a food diary for a few days, including both weekdays and weekends, to help identify your eating patterns. Be sure to note the time of each meal or snack so you can see how frequently you eat. Don't forget to record the amount of fluids you drink during the day. All of this information can help you identify where to start making changes in your eating plan.

Step 3: Decide When and How to Start

Success is important when you are trying something new or making any kind of change. This is especially true when it comes to eating. If you are successful at the beginning, you will be more likely to stick with your new habits and to feel motivated to make more changes as needed. Therefore, it is wise to look ahead to identify the factors that will help you make the changes you want, as well as the factors that will make it difficult to change. For example, consider the following types of questions:

- Is there someone or something that will make it easier to change?
- Will worries or concerns about friends, work, or other commitments affect your ability to follow through?

Food Diary			
Time of Meal/Snack	*What You Ate*	*How Much (size of portion)*	*Number of Servings for Each Food Group*
			__protein __vegetable __dairy __fruit __starch __fats & sweets
			__protein __vegetable __dairy __fruit __starch __fats & sweets
			__protein __vegetable __dairy __fruit __starch __fats & sweets
			__protein __vegetable __dairy __fruit __starch __fats & sweets
			__protein __vegetable __dairy __fruit __starch __fats & sweets
			__protein __vegetable __dairy __fruit __starch __fats & sweets

Totals: __protein __starch __fruit
__dairy __vegetable __fats & sweets

- How can you coordinate your medications with food?
- How will medications affect your appetite?
- Are there obstacles that will keep you from changing the way you eat?

Examine all these factors. Then find ways to build support for the desired changes or to minimize any problems you anticipate. Once you have done this, set the date on which you will begin to make your changes. If you decide that it is too difficult to start making those changes now, set a date in the future to reevaluate your plan. In the meantime, accept that this is the right decision for you, and focus your attention on other goals. You do not have to change everything at once. Remember, slow and steady wins the race.

When you are ready, begin with the changes that are easiest. Make one change at a time. You may decide to change how often you eat before changing what you eat. If you skip meals now, it might be a good idea to start by eating more regularly. After you get into the habit of eating four or more times a day, you might make other changes, such as adding more vegetables and fruits to your eating plan, or eating more breads and cereals.

Use the action plan discussed in Chapter 2 to help you incorporate these changes into your daily routine. Following are ideas to help you overcome some of the problems many of us encounter when trying to change our eating habits.

Dealing with Problems in Changing Eating Habits

I eat out a lot, so how do I know if I'm eating well?

Whether it's because you don't have enough time, hate to cook, or just don't have the energy to go grocery shopping and prepare meals, eating out may suit your needs. This is not necessarily bad, if you know which choices are healthy ones. These tips may help:

- Select restaurants that not only serve a variety of dishes but also offer variety in the way they prepare those dishes. Nowadays many restaurants, even some fast-food chains, offer nutritious food choices. For example, you can choose a dish that is grilled or broiled rather than fried, or a salad and baked potato instead of a hamburger and fries.

- Ask what is in a dish and how it is prepared, especially if it is a dish you have not tried before.

- Choose restaurants that list ingredients on their menus. That way, you can order dishes that are right for your special needs, whether you are trying to increase protein or fiber, reduce fat, add calories, or limit carbohydrates.

- Follow the food safety guidelines for eating out (see p. 187).

I know some foods are good for me, but I just don't like them.

If you don't like a certain food, try substituting another food in the same food group. If you don't like an entire food group, you may need to consult with a nutritionist to find foods from other groups that can give you similar nutrients.

I don't like vegetables.

Try raw vegetables with tasty dips or sauces to add flavor. Grated or frozen vegetables can be used in soups, stews, or meat loaf. Try vegetable casseroles, such as vegetable lasagna. If vegetables still don't appeal to you, increase the amounts of fruits and breads you eat.

I don't like to drink milk.

Instead of drinking milk, add it (or dry milk powder) to foods such as soups, meat loaf, or casseroles. You can also choose pudding, yogurt, cottage cheese, or ice cream in place of milk. Try yogurt in a salad dressing or in a vegetable or fruit dip. Melt some cheese on vegetables, on potatoes, on beans, on tortillas, in sandwiches, on pizza, or in a dip. To get some of the same nutrients that are in milk without eating cheese or yogurt, try broccoli, greens (such as kale or collard or beet greens), tofu, beans, canned salmon, and corn tortillas. If milk or milk products make you feel bloated and cause diarrhea or gas, see the discussion of dairy products and lactose intolerance on page 177.

I'm a vegetarian. I don't want to eat any animal foods.

You can be a vegetarian and still have a healthy eating plan. To make sure you get the protein and other nutrients usually supplied by food from animals, include fortified soybean milk, tofu, beans, and other plant protein sources along with a variety of breads, grains, pasta, fruits, and vegetables. If meat, fish, and poultry are the only animal foods you don't eat, include a variety of dairy products and eggs.

I eat when I'm feeling bored, depressed, lonely, or otherwise discontent.

Many people find comfort in food. Some people eat when they don't have anything else to do. Some eat when they're feeling down or bothered. Unfortunately, at these times you may lose track of what and how much you eat. These are also times when "healthy" foods, such as fruits and vegetables, never seem to do the trick. The following strategies can help:

- Keep track of your eating patterns. List what, how much, and when you eat. Note how you are feeling when you have the urge to eat. Try to spot patterns.

- Make a plan for when these situations arise. If you catch yourself feeling bored or down in the dumps, try to do something else instead of eating "junk" food. Do some light exercise, practice a relaxation or distraction technique, or engage in your favorite hobby.

I'd rather eat sweets and snack foods such as chips, candy, and cookies.

You can include these foods in your meals and snacks; in fact, they are important sources of calories. But try to eat foods from each of the primary food groups first. If you're still hungry or if you have a taste for more, then add your favorite sweets and snack foods. Try not to let chips, candy, and cookies take the place of other foods that are more nutritious.

It takes too long to prepare meals. By the time I'm done, I'm too tired to eat!

You need to eat to maintain your energy level. If meal preparation is a problem for you, it's time to develop a plan. Here are some energy-saving suggestions:

- Plan your meals for the week. Then go to the grocery store and buy everything you will need.
- Break your food preparation into steps, resting in between.
- Cook enough for two, three, or even more servings, especially if it's something you really like.
- Freeze the extra portions in single-serving sizes. On the days when you are really tired, thaw and reheat one of these precooked frozen meals.
- Ask for help, especially for big meals or at social gatherings.

I've never really been a cook, and I can't start now.

Keep it simple. Keep your freezer stocked with prepared meals: pizzas, vegetables, and other convenience foods. Try easy-to-prepare meals such as a grilled cheese sandwich and canned soup, eggs and toast, cereal and milk, or macaroni and cheese. Go to the library or a bookstore and look through some cookbooks to get ideas for quick meals. When you do cook, make larger amounts and freeze portions to reheat later.

Managing Specific Eating Problems

Like everyone, you want to eat healthy food that tastes good and makes you feel good. But having HIV may create specific eating problems that are not as common in other people. The symptoms you experience from an infection, from depression, or as medication side effects often affect how you feel about eating. The result can be weight loss, which weakens the body's ability to fight off other illnesses. Some medications can cause other conditions, such as high cholesterol and high blood sugar (hyperglycemia or even diabetes), which may require even more changes in your eating plan. Eating a variety of foods and maintaining a healthy weight are important goals for the person with HIV; therefore, it is necessary to find ways to deal with some of the specific problems that interfere with your eating. Let's look at some of these problems.

I don't feel like eating anything.

Loss of appetite is a common problem that can be caused by medication, fatigue, concern about your illness, or an infection. On days when you feel like eating, be sure to eat plenty to make up for days when your appetite is bad. When you are having trouble with poor appetite, the following suggestions can help you get the calories you need.

- Eat smaller meals more frequently (six times a day).
- Eat in a relaxed setting, with a friend, or while listening to your favorite music.
- Eat your favorite foods as often as you like, even if it is just a little bit.
- Add more flavor to your foods with spices and herbs, lemon wedges, mustard, barbecue sauce, catsup, or hot sauce.
- Have take-out food delivered to your home, or check in your area for home food-delivery services, such as Project Open Hand or Meals on Wheels.
- Keep a supply of high-calorie, high-protein snacks on hand, such as crackers, cheese, peanut butter, and ice cream. Eat these whenever you feel like it.
- Try liquid foods or foods that do not take a lot of energy to chew or cook. When you don't feel like eating much, make a milk shake or have a supplement drink. (Your doctor, nurse, or nutritionist can recommend one.)

- Avoid filling up on liquids before you eat. Drink small amounts when you eat, and sip fluids between your eating times.
- Keep easy-to-prepare foods on hand, such as canned food, frozen meals, or frozen leftovers.
- Pack nonperishable food to snack on when you are away from home. Keep snacks in handy places around the house—for example, near your bedside or where you relax at home.
- Do light exercise before you eat to help increase your appetite.
- Ask your doctor about medications or natural remedies that can stimulate your appetite, especially if you seem to be losing weight.

It's important to eat enough calories and nutrients to avoid weight loss. If you find that you can't keep your appetite up, consult your doctor. He or she can refer you to a nutritionist, who can help you plan meals that maximize the value of what you eat.

I get full too fast.

Eat often during the day. Three meals a day may not be enough for you, especially if you can't eat a full meal at one sitting. Eating five or six times per day seems to work best for most people with HIV/AIDS, particularly those who do not feel well. Make what you eat count: choose foods with lots of calories and protein to help meet your needs for these important nutrients.

Food doesn't taste as good as before.

Oral infections, such as thrush, and certain medications can change your taste sensations, as well as your ability to enjoy food. You may also experience a bitter or metallic taste in your mouth. The following suggestions can help you manage this problem and enhance the flavor of food.

- Rinse your mouth with a mixture of 1 teaspoon of hydrogen peroxide or baking soda in a glass of warm distilled water before eating. Swish the mixture around in your mouth, but do not swallow. Also, if oral or esophageal thrush is a problem for you, remember to take your antifungal medication to prevent it.
- Use flavored toothpaste on a soft-bristled toothbrush to clean your teeth and tongue before and after you eat.
- To mask the metallic taste, try drinking orange, cranberry, or pineapple juice; lemonade; or another tart drink.

- Modify recipes to include a variety of ingredients that make your food look and taste more appealing. Add vinegar, lemon juice, pickles, or fresh and dried herbs to your food. Start with about ¼ teaspoon of herbs (rosemary, thyme, basil, oregano, cilantro, cumin) in a dish that serves four. Try adding chopped nuts or seeds to your food; this gives the food a different texture and makes eating a bit more interesting.

Getting More Calories and Protein

Add:	*To:*
Butter, margarine, sour cream	Vegetables, cooked cereal, potatoes, noodles, or rice
Dried fruits or nuts, honey, jelly, jam, syrup, sugar, cream, half-and-half, yogurt	Hot or cold cereal, pancakes, or waffles
Bacon, avocado, olives, mayonnaise, salad dressing	Sandwiches, salads, or casseroles
Cream or sour cream	Soups, fruit, or puddings
Cheese or cream cheese	Fruit or crackers
Peanut butter or other nut butter	Sauces, shakes, toast, crackers, waffles, fresh fruit, or raw vegetables
Chopped meat; canned tuna, salmon, shrimp, or crab meat; shredded cheese; hard-cooked eggs; egg substitutes; beans; tofu	Soups, sauces, vegetables, salads, or casseroles
Gravy	Meat, poultry, or potatoes
Honey, sugar, molasses, syrup	Milk shakes, hot or cold tea, Kool-Aid, or lemonade
Dried fruit, syrup	Ice cream, yogurt, or frozen yogurt
Dry milk powder	Regular milk, scrambled eggs, soups, gravies, or desserts

- Marinate meat, poultry, fish, or tofu in vinegar, wine, salad dressing, or soy sauce.
- Eat cold foods such as sherbet, fruit ice, frozen yogurt, and ice cream to numb your taste buds.
- Chew your food well so that it will remain in your mouth longer to stimulate your taste buds.

When I eat, I feel like I'm going to throw up.

An infection or a medication side effect can cause nausea, making foods unappealing. The following suggestions may help you to manage these symptoms.

- Eat smaller, snack-sized meals throughout the day. Often nausea is worse when the stomach is empty
- Drink high-calorie fluids one hour after eating, not during meals.
- Avoid spicy and fatty foods, as well as caffeine. These can irritate the stomach and intestines.
- Eat cold, blander-tasting foods such as ice cream, frozen yogurt, gelatin, pudding or custard, cottage cheese and fruit, juice, cold cereal, or a sandwich. These may be easier to take.
- Try salty or dry foods, such as bread or crackers. These may help calm your stomach.
- Rest between meals, but do not lie completely flat. Elevate your upper body or sit up for at least two hours after eating.
- If the smell of food bothers you, ask someone else to cook for you or make sure that the cooking area is well ventilated so that food smells don't linger.
- Avoid eating your favorite foods when you feel sick, so that you don't start to associate them with nausea and dislike them later.
- Drink a cup of herbal tea (chamomile or peppermint) with honey or a piece of fresh ginger added, or chew on a piece of fresh ginger root to help settle your stomach.
- If your medication seems to cause nausea, talk to your doctor or a pharmacist about timing your doses so that you take them when you are eating or right after you eat.

- Ask your doctor about taking antinausea medication. If one medication doesn't work, ask for a stronger one. Take the medication as directed, which is typically a half hour before meals.

Diarrhea is a problem for me.

Diarrhea can be caused by many things, including medications, stress, infections, or severe weight loss. Whatever the cause, diarrhea means that your body is not getting the fluids and nutrients it needs from the foods you eat. For this reason, it is critical that you pay attention to your fluid intake to prevent dehydration.

The following tips will help you deal with and lessen your diarrhea.

- Drink high-calorie fluids (at least eight glasses per day), such as juices, clear carbonated beverages, broth, and fruit or sports drinks. Water should not be the only thing you drink, because it lacks the calories and nutrients your body must replace. Avoid drinks that have caffeine or alcohol; these stimulate the intestines and can cause further dehydration. Try frozen liquids such as ice pops or sherbet, but eat or drink these at room temperature. Very hot or cold fluids may stimulate the intestines and make diarrhea worse.

- Potassium is a vital mineral that is lost when you have diarrhea, and depletion can lead to muscle cramping and fatigue. Replace lost potassium by eating bananas, raisins, sports drinks, fruit juices (especially orange juice and nectars), vegetable juices, mashed potatoes, or canned fruits without seeds or skins.

- You may not feel like eating much, but skipping meals is not a good idea. Foods you may be able to tolerate are plain white rice, noodles, mashed potatoes, crackers, white toast, eggs, hot cereal, applesauce or other canned fruits without seeds or skins, bananas, gelatin, ice cream, sherbet, or broth-type soups.

- Avoid greasy or fatty foods that have large amounts of butter, margarine, or oils, and foods that are fried. For more tips, see the following discussion of fat intolerance.

- Avoid foods that are high in fiber or that have skins or seeds; these can be irritating and hard to digest. Avoid raw fruits and vegetables and whole-grain breads or cereals. Low-fiber foods, such as cooked vegetables, canned fruits without skins or seeds, ripe bananas, white rice, and white bread, are good choices.

- Avoid milk or milk products for a while. Drink low-fat milk and eat lean meats if you can tolerate them. Dairy aids containing lactase can help you digest and absorb the milk sugar that causes some people problems such as bloating and diarrhea (see the following discussion of lactose intolerance). Stick to plain boiled, baked, or broiled meats, and stay away from spicy foods or sauces.

- Cramps often accompany diarrhea and can be a sign of gas or air in your intestines. Carbonated beverages can worsen this problem and should be avoided. Foods that cause gas, such as raw apples, beans, cabbage, broccoli, cauliflower, onions, green peppers, and beer, should also be avoided.

- Ask your doctor about antidiarrheal medications. A tablespoon of Metamucil mixed with juice also may help control diarrhea, because the soluble fiber in it makes the stool bulky.

Note: If your diarrhea increases in frequency or lasts for more than a week, consult your doctor. Unchecked diarrhea can cause further problems, and medications to help you get it under control are available. Dehydration and potassium loss are the serious problems that must be prevented or corrected. (See Chapter 7 for more information about evaluating diarrhea.)

What if I am constipated?

Constipation is often the result of not drinking enough fluids, not eating enough food or fiber, and not being physically active. Constipation may also develop as a side effect of certain medications, especially narcotic-based pain medications. In addition to drinking enough fluids, try these suggestions:

- Eat foods high in insoluble fiber, such as whole-grain breads and cereals, fresh fruits and vegetables, cooked beans and chickpeas, nuts, and seeds.

- Add small amounts of bran to food or liquids, to increase fiber.

- Include some aerobic exercise in your daily schedule.

- Ask your doctor about medications to relieve constipation.

I have trouble digesting fat (fat intolerance).

Fats are an excellent source of calories. They can also be hard to digest. Fat intolerance—difficulty digesting and absorbing fats—can be a problem for people with HIV infection and AIDS. If you feel discomfort after eating foods high

Foods High in Fat

- Fried foods
- Chips
- Tuna in oil
- French fries
- Salad dressing
- Chocolate
- Rich desserts
- Too much butter, oil, or margarine

- Mayonnaise
- Pepperoni
- Cheeses
- Cream sauces
- Hot dogs
- Ice cream
- Sausages
- Cream or half-and-half

- Whole milk
- Luncheon meats
- Bacon
- Gravies
- Peanut butter
- Doughnuts

in fat, you may need to reduce the amount of fat you eat. It is not usually a good idea to completely eliminate fat, unless you are experiencing prolonged and severe diarrhea. If fat intolerance becomes a chronic problem, it is best to avoid fat-rich foods, such the ones listed in the accompanying table.

If your problem with fat is severe, products that contain no fat but have extra calories and protein are available. Other products have a special, easily digestible form of fat. These products may be help you to keep your intake and weight at appropriate levels.

I don't feel well when I eat dairy products (lactose intolerance).

If you notice that milk, cheese, and ice cream cause cramping, gas, bloating, or diarrhea, your body may be having trouble digesting lactose, a type of sugar found in milk and milk products. If your reactions subside with time, you can start eating these dairy foods again. After all, they are good protein sources.

The following suggestions can help you avoid the more troublesome dairy products and find ones that you are able to tolerate.

- Avoid foods containing milk, such as pudding, custard, ice cream, cream soups, cream pies, gravies, and sauces.

- Use milk and milk products that contain an enzyme called *lactase,* which will help you digest lactose. Such items are found in the regular dairy section of your supermarket. Check the labels before buying.

- Some dairy products contain less lactose and therefore may be easier to tolerate. These include buttermilk, cottage cheese, sour cream, aged cheeses, sherbet, and yogurt. In place of milk, try nondairy products like enriched soy milk, nondairy cream, or other milk substitutes.

- Kosher foods labeled *pareve* or *parve* are acceptable because they are milk free.

- Use lactase pills or drops before eating something that has large amounts of lactose.

Dry mouth, mouth sores, and swallowing problems make it hard to eat anything.

Your mouth may feel dry as a side effect of some medications or from not drinking enough fluids. Also, infections in your mouth and throat can cause sores that make it painful to eat or swallow. The following tips may help you manage these symptoms.

- Avoid smoking or drinking alcohol; these irritate the mouth and throat.

- Soft foods that are smooth in consistency and easy to swallow are usually the easiest to eat. You can make swallowing easier by putting food through a blender, eating casseroles and stews, or adding butter, gravy, sauce, or salad dressing to moisten food. Choose dishes that don't have chunks of food in them. Add liquids to foods or dunk foods in soup, milk, juice, or hot chocolate. This makes them less irritating to your mouth and throat.

- Avoid spicy foods, foods with a high acid content (such as orange juice or tomatoes), and carbonated sodas. These can make mouth sores burn. Cold foods such as ice pops, ice cream, sherbet, frozen yogurt, or thick milk shakes can numb your mouth and are easy to swallow.

- If you find that you gag easily, avoid sticky foods, such as peanut butter, and slippery foods, such as gelatin.

- Use a straw for drinking fluids and a cup or glass for eating soup. Tilt your head back to make swallowing easier.

- Try eating soft, bland foods such as pudding, custard, eggs, canned fruits, cottage cheese, yogurt, bananas, and creamed cereals.

- Avoid foods that require a lot of chewing or are tough and fibrous.
- Suck on sugar-free candy or sour hard candy, popsicles, or ice, or chew sugarless gum to stimulate salivation.
- Rinse your mouth frequently and drink lots of fluids to help with dryness. If dryness continues to be a problem even when you moisten your foods, your doctor or dentist may prescribe artificial saliva for you.
- Sleep with a humidifier in your room, and keep fluids by your bedside to sip on during the night if you are thirsty.

What if I Have Other Health Problems?

Some eating tips are important for people with HIV/AIDS who have developed diabetes or high cholesterol as a result of taking certain medications. The following information may help you control these conditions and prevent further complications.

Diabetes

If you have diabetes, it is important to watch the amount of carbohydrates you eat. Carbohydrates (starches and sugars) are the nutrients that break down into glucose. With the help of a hormone called *insulin,* the glucose is able to pass from the blood stream into the body's cells, to be used as energy. When you have diabetes, however, either the body does not produce enough insulin or the cells cannot use the insulin produced. This means that the glucose stays in the blood stream and can cause complications. For this reason, we recommend that you limit the amount of foods you eat that are high in carbohydrates and that you eat equal-size meals every four to five hours during the day.

The recommended amount of carbohydrates for each meal is 45 to 60 grams, equal to about three to four servings of foods that are rich in carbohydrates, such as the starchy vegetables (potatoes, corn, beets, peas), breads, rice, pasta, and fruit. Each of these foods contains approximately 15 grams of carbohydrate per portion. Most other vegetables are low in carbohydrates; these can usually be eaten in unlimited quantities because they contain only about 5 grams of carbohydrates per recommended serving. Other foods that should be limited include sweets (cakes, cookies, ice cream, etc.) and alcohol.

Although meat, fish, and poultry are low in carbohydrates, they do contain fat; therefore, we do not recommend exceeding the suggested portion size and number of servings per day (2 to 3 ounces, three times per day).

People with diabetes have an increased risk of developing heart disease, circulatory problems, and high blood pressure. For this reason, it is important to reduce the fat, cholesterol, and sodium (salt) in the foods you eat. This, along with regular exercise, can help lower your blood sugar.

High Cholesterol

If you have high cholesterol or high triglycerides (fats in the blood), it is a good idea to reduce the amount of fat and cholesterol you eat and to increase your fiber intake. Avoid the fatty foods listed on page 177, and look at the following hints for reducing fat and increasing fiber. These tips will help you to prevent the narrowing and hardening of the arteries that can cause heart attacks, and to control your blood pressure, blood sugar, and weight.

If you also have high blood pressure (hypertension), eat less salt and sodium. Read nutrition labels for sodium content, and experiment with herbs and spices to season your food. Unfortunately, many prepackaged, processed

Hints for Reducing Fat in Your Eating Plan

- Eat more poultry and fish, and less red meat (limit portions to 2–3 oz or 50–100 g, about the size of a deck of cards).
- Choose leaner cuts of meat.
- Trim the yellow fat and remove the skin from poultry.
- Eat egg yolks and organ meats (liver, kidneys, brains) in moderation.
- Broil, barbecue, or roast meats instead of frying them.
- Avoid deep-fat-fried foods.
- Skim fat off stews and soups.
- Use low- or nonfat milk and milk products.
- Use fats such as butter, margarine, oils, gravy, sauces, and salad dressings sparingly (no more than 3 to 4 teaspoons or 15–20 ml per day).
- Use a nonstick pan with cooking oil spray.

Hints for Increasing Fiber in Your Eating Plan

- Build your meals around vegetables, grain products, and fruits.
- Eat a variety of fruits and vegetables, raw or lightly cooked.
- Eat low-fat grain products such as whole-wheat breads, brown rice, and corn tortillas.
- Eat more lentils or beans and rice and less meat.
- Snack on fruit or nonfat yogurt, not sweets or ice cream.
- Drink plenty of water to help move the fiber through your system.

foods are high in sugar, fat, and sodium. If you use these foods often, choose the brands that are lowest in sugar, fat, and sodium.

If you are dealing with diabetes or high cholesterol, be sure to consult a nutritionist to help determine the best eating plan for you. You may also need other medications to help control these problems.

Changing your eating habits is not easy, and the suggestions given here are only a start. But the key to changing how you eat is the overall approach: make sure you're motivated, figure out what you're doing now, figure out some practical changes you can make, and solve any problems that come up. These steps really can be applied to all kinds of changes you might want to make, and good self-managers use them all the time.

Suggested Reading

American Dietetic Association. *Living Well with HIV and AIDS: A Guide to Healthy Eating.* Chicago: American Dietetic Association, 1993.

Brody, Jane. *Jane Brody's Nutrition Book.* New York: Bantam Doubleday, 1989.

Deutsch, Ronald M., and Morrill, Judi S. *Realities of Nutrition.* Palo Alto, CA: Bull Publishing, 1993.

Ferguson, James M. *Habits Not Diets.* 2nd ed. Palo Alto, CA: Bull Publishing, 1988.

Lappé, Frances. *Diet for a Small Planet.* 20th anniversary ed. New York: Ballantine, 1992.

Robertson, Laurel, Ruppenthal, Brian, and Flinders, Carol. *Laurel's Kitchen Caring: Recipes for Everyday Home Caregiving.* Berkeley: Ten Speed Press, 1997.

Robertson, Laurel, Ruppenthal, Brian, and Flinders, Carol. *The New Laurel's Kitchen: A Handbook for Vegetarian Cookery and Nutrition.* Berkeley: Ten Speed Press, 1986.

12   Food Safety and Preparation Tips

Just as you need to eat well when you have HIV disease, you must also protect yourself from bacteria that can cause food poisoning. People with HIV/AIDS are more likely than people with strong immune systems to acquire food-borne illnesses that can be hard to treat.

Food poisoning can cause nausea, vomiting, and diarrhea, all of which will make you miserable and interfere with your eating. This, in turn, leads to weight loss, further weakens your immune system, and hastens the progression of the disease.

Since most food contamination results from the improper handling of food, you can protect yourself by following some basic safety guidelines when buying, preparing, serving, and storing foods. These guidelines are also important to keep in mind when eating away from home or traveling abroad. The American Dietetic Association recommends the following precautions for safety.

Shopping for food

- Read food labels carefully. Avoid products that contain raw or undercooked meat and dairy products. Avoid all dairy products that are not pasteurized.
- Check the dates on food packages. Don't buy or use packaged food that has passed the recommended date on the label.
- Don't buy food with damaged packaging or food that has been handled or displayed improperly.
- Put packaged meat, poultry, or fish into a plastic bag before placing it in your shopping cart.
- Shop for cold and frozen foods last, and ask that these foods be packed in the same bag.

- Carry a cooler in your car to store the cold and frozen foods if the trip home takes longer than thirty minutes.
- Check your refrigerator regularly and throw away foods that are past the expiration date.

Food storage

- Storing foods properly is the key to food safety. Be sure to refrigerate or freeze foods that require cold storage as soon as possible after buying them. The temperature in your refrigerator should be 40°F or lower, and the freezer temperature should be 0°F or lower. Use a refrigerator thermometer to make sure temperatures are in the proper range.
- Label your stored foods with the date of purchase, and follow the recommended storage times for each type of food. Foods that contain harmful bacteria do not always look or smell spoiled. When in doubt, throw it out.
- Always thaw frozen foods in the refrigerator or microwave oven. Do not allow drippings from defrosting foods (especially meat, poultry, or fish) to touch other foods in the refrigerator. Place them in a separate container on the bottom shelf of the refrigerator to thaw.
- Put leftover prepared foods containing meat, eggs, or milk products in the refrigerator or freezer immediately. Store the portions in small containers for easy use later.
- Cover food tightly with plastic wrap or in airtight containers.
- Don't eat leftovers that have been in the refrigerator for more than two days.

Food preparation and cooking

- Always begin by washing your hands with soapy water. Remember to wash your hands again after handling any raw foods and before handling cooked food.
- Don't use wooden cutting boards for meat, poultry, or fish; plastic boards are easier to sanitize.
- Clean all utensils, plastic cutting boards, and chipped china or crockery in the dishwasher, or wash them in hot, soapy water (at least 140°F) and rinse them well.

Refrigerated Products Stored at 35° to 40°F

Food Product	Use Within:
• Raw beefsteaks and roasts, raw pork chops, raw lamb chops and roasts, cooked ham, lunch meat	3–5 days
• Ground beef, turkey, pork, or lamb; sausage	1–2 days
• Hot dogs	1 week
• Raw chicken or turkey, giblets, fish	1–2 days
• Leftover cooked meat and meat dishes; soups and stews	3–4 days
• Leftover gravy and meat broth	1–2 days
• Leftover cooked poultry and poultry dishes	3–4 days
• Leftover cooked poultry covered with broth or gravy; leftover chicken nuggets, patties, or fried chicken	1–2 days
• Fresh eggs in the shell	3 weeks
• Raw yolks or whites (out of the shell)	2–4 days
• Hard-cooked eggs	1 week

- Sanitize your plastic cutting board after working with raw meats, fish, and poultry. Soak the board in a solution of 1–2 tablespoons of bleach per gallon of warm water for ten minutes.
- Clean utensils, countertops, shelves, refrigerator, and freezer with this same bleach solution as an additional safety step.
- Keep towels and sponges clean. Replace sponges often, and use different sponges for washing dishes and for other types of cleaning.

Meat, poultry, and fish

- Never eat raw meat, poultry, or fish of any kind. Even steak tartare, carpaccio, raw oysters, raw shrimp, sashimi, or sushi topped with raw fish can cause serious infections.

- Cook all meats to 165°F or higher. Cook poultry to 180°F. Use a meat thermometer to check the temperature.

- Cook all meats completely. Red meat should be well done, and poultry should be cooked until the juices are clear.

- Reheat all leftovers thoroughly, to 165°F or higher.

- When barbecuing, precook meats just before putting them on the grill to make sure that the inside reaches the proper temperature.

- Eat meats and meat dishes while they are hot, and store leftovers in the refrigerator immediately. Don't let them sit out at room temperature for more than two hours.

Eggs

- Check at the store to make sure you don't buy eggs with cracked shells. Refrigerate eggs as soon as you get home. Never let eggs or dishes prepared with eggs sit out at room temperature.

- Don't eat raw eggs or eggs that are soft-boiled, or scrambled but runny. Avoid foods prepared with uncooked or undercooked eggs, such as Caesar salad dressing, chocolate mousse, some frostings, homemade eggnog, and homemade mayonnaise. If you eat homemade ice cream, check to see if raw eggs are an ingredient.

- When cooking eggs, make sure the yolk and white are firm. Follow these cooking times and temperatures:
  - *Scrambled eggs:* Cook for 1 minute at medium setting (250°F for electric frying pans).
  - *Sunny-side-up eggs:* Cook for 7 minutes at medium setting (250°F), or cook covered for 4 minutes at 250°F.
  - *Fried, over-easy eggs:* Cook for 3 minutes at medium setting on one side, then for 1 minute on the other side.
  - *Poached eggs:* Cook for 5 minutes in boiling water.
  - *Hard-boiled eggs:* Cook for at least 7 minutes in boiling water.

- If a recipe calls for raw eggs and the mixture will not be cooked, use a pasteurized, frozen egg product instead.

Milk and dairy products

- Buy only pasteurized milk and dairy products. Read the labels on cheeses, as not all of them are pasteurized.
- Check the expiration date. Buy products before the expiration date, and use them within the next several days.
- Don't eat soft-ripened cheeses or cheese that has mold on it. Throw away moldy cheese.

Fruits and vegetables

- Choose fresh fruits and vegetables with unbroken skins.
- Wash all fruits and vegetables thoroughly and peel those with skin.
- Avoid fruits and vegetables that are moldy or have soft spots that show signs of rotting or mold.
- Refrigerate to reduce spoilage.

Eating out

- Be sure your eating utensils, place settings, and beverage glasses are clean. Don't be shy about returning dirty utensils or food that is not hot enough or not cooked thoroughly.
- In a restaurant avoid eating the same foods that you avoid eating at home.
- Avoid salad bars. You can't be sure how well the vegetables or fruits have been washed or handled, or how long they have been sitting out. If you are given a choice between salad and soup, choose the soup.
- Order meats medium-well to well done. To check doneness, cut into the center of the meat. If it is pink or bloody, it needs to be cooked more. Fish should be flaky, not rubbery, when cut.
- Order eggs cooked on both sides, and don't eat runny-looking eggs.
- If you are not sure about the ingredients and preparation of a dish, ask before ordering.
- Don't eat raw or even lightly steamed seafood.

Traveling abroad

- Boil all water before drinking.
- Drink only beverages made with boiled water, and canned or carbonated bottled drinks. Use only ice cubes that have been made from boiled water.
- Avoid uncooked vegetables and salads.
- Peel all fruit.
- Eat cooked foods while they are still hot.

While for most people food poisoning can be treated with rest and plenty of fluids, this is not true for people with HIV or AIDS. They may experience more serious and prolonged symptoms that are difficult to treat. They will require a doctor's care.

After reading this chapter, you might feel that just because you have HIV, eating has become a big, complicated hassle. Luckily, it doesn't have to be that way. It is true that you may need to modify what you eat and follow some basic food safety guidelines, but such changes are not always difficult. In fact, these are safety measures that everyone should practice. With a little thought and planning, mealtime can be one of the best parts of your day. Eating healthfully and safely will allow you to enjoy your food even more!

Managing Personal and Practical Issues

13   Communicating

Y*ou just don't understand!* How often has this statement, expressed or unexpressed, summed up a frustrating verbal exchange? The goal in any communication between you and another is, first, that the other person understand what you are trying to say. Feeling that you are not understood leads to frustration, and a prolonged feeling of frustration can lead to depression, anger, and helplessness. These are not good feelings for anyone, especially people with chronic illness. Dealing with HIV/AIDS can be frustrating enough without adding communication problems.

Poor communication is the biggest factor in poor relationships, whether they be between spouses, family members or friends, coworkers, or doctors and patients. (For a discussion on communication with your doctor, see pages 43–46.) Even in casual relationships, poor communication causes frustration. How often have you been angry and frustrated as a customer, and how often is this because of poor communication?

When you have a chronic illness, good communication becomes a necessity. As a self-manager, it is in your best interest to learn the skills necessary to make the communications in your life the most effective possible. In this chapter, we discuss ways to improve the communication process: how to express feelings in a positive way, how to ask for help, how to say "no," how to listen, and how to get more information from the other person.

While reading this chapter, keep in mind that *communication is a two-way street.* As uncomfortable as you may feel about expressing your feelings and asking for help, chances are that others are also feeling this way. It may be up to you to make sure the lines of communication are open.

Verbalizing Feelings: "I" Messages

Let's face it, many of us are uncomfortable expressing our feelings, especially if doing so means we might seem critical of the person we're talking to. Yet when emotions are high, attempts to express frustration can be laden with *"you" messages. You* can be an accusatory word, suggesting blame. Its use, when expressing feelings, can cause the other person to feel as though he or she is under attack. Suddenly, the other person feels on the defensive, and protective barriers go up. The person trying to express feelings, in turn, feels greater anxiety, and the situation escalates to anger, frustration, and bad feelings.

I, on the other hand, is not an accusatory word. It doesn't strike out or blame. When expressing your own feelings, express them in terms of how *you* feel, not how the other person *makes* you feel.

Following are some examples of "you" and "I" messages.

"You" Message Example

Partner 1:   You never seem to be interested in sex anymore. I wish you would just try to show some interest.

Partner 2:   You seem to have nothing else on your mind but sex. I just have so many other things to worry about right now . . . juggling my meds, exercising, eating right.

Partner 1:   But what about my needs? Why don't you make that one of your priorities? You're being very self-centered.

Partner 2:   ME self-centered? All you think about is sex, and you're calling me self-centered!?!

Partner 1:   Well, I can see once again that talking about this is getting us nowhere. It just makes it all worse!

"I" Message Example

Partner 1:   I really miss having sex with you. It's been awhile, hasn't it?

Partner 2:   Yes, it has. I just feel so overwhelmed with trying to adjust to the medication schedules and doctor appointments, and trying to focus on staying healthy, that I don't have as much energy as I used to.

Partner 1:	I never really thought about how much more complicated your life has become with all the new pills you're taking. Still, I miss feeling close and intimate. Having sex always helped me feel closer to you.
Partner 2:	I really miss that, too, but I just don't have the energy for having sex. I feel tired most of the time.
Partner 1:	Maybe if we just spend some time alone holding each other and talking, that will help me feel close to you again.
Partner 2:	That would really feel great. I miss cuddling with you at night, but I didn't want to make you think I was initiating sex. If we can just hold each other, that would be a big load off my mind.
Partner 1:	That sounds like a great compromise to me. And maybe we can come up with some ideas of how I can help you with the details in your life.

The trick to "I" messages is to avoid the use of the word *you* and to instead report your personal feelings using the word *I*. Of course, like any new skill, "I"

"I" Message Exercise

Change the following statements into "I" messages. (Watch out for hidden "you" messages!) When you have finished the exercise, compare your "I" messages with our suggestions at the bottom of the page.

1. You expect me to wait on you hand and foot!

2. You hardly ever touch me anymore. You don't pay any attention to me since I tested positive.

3. You don't tell me the side effects of all these drugs you're giving me or why I have to take them, doctor.

Sample answers to "I" Messages Exercise above:

1. I'm frustrated by your illness. I feel as though I'm doing more than my share right now.

2. I'm concerned that we seem to have grown apart since I tested positive.

3. I don't feel well informed about the drugs I'm taking, doctor. *Or:* I feel I need to understand more about the medications I'm taking.

messages take practice. Start by really listening, both to yourself and to others. Take some of the "you" messages you hear and turn them into "I" messages in your head. By playing this little word game in your head, you'll be surprised at how fast "I" messages become a habit in your own expressions.

There are some cautions to note when using "I" messages. First, they are not a miracle cure. Sometimes the listener has to have time to hear them. This is especially true if "you" messages and blaming have been the more usual ways of communicating. Even if at first using "I" messages seems ineffective, continue to use them and refine your skill. Some people may use "I" messages as a means of manipulation. If used in this way, problems can escalate. To be used effectively, "I" messages must report *honest* feelings.

Note: "I" messages are an excellent way to express *positive* feelings and compliments! "I really appreciate the extra time you gave me today."

Asking for Help

Problems with communication about the subject of help are pretty common. For some reason, people feel awkward about asking for help or refusing help. Although this problem is probably universal, it can come up more often for people with HIV/AIDS.

It may be emotionally difficult for some of us to ask for needed help. Maybe it's difficult for us to admit to ourselves that we are unable to do things as easily as in the past. When this is the case, try to avoid hedging your request with: "I'm sorry to have to ask this . . . ," "I know this is asking a lot . . . ," "I hate to ask this, but . . ." Hedging tends to put the other person on the defensive ("Gosh, what's he going to ask for that's so much, anyway?"). Be specific about what help you are requesting. A general request can lead to misunderstanding, and the other person can react negatively to insufficient information.

General request:	"I know this is the last thing you want to do, but I need help moving. Will you help me?"
Reaction:	"Uh . . . well . . . I don't know. Um . . . can I get back to you after I check my schedule?" (Probably next year!)
Specific request:	"I'm moving next week, and I'd like to move my books and kitchen stuff ahead of time. Would you mind helping me load and unload the boxes in my

	car Saturday morning? I think it can be done in one trip."
Reaction:	"I'm busy Saturday morning, but I could give you a hand Friday night, if you'd like."

People with chronic illness must also sometimes deal with offers of help that are not needed or desired. In most cases, these offers come from people who are dear to you and genuinely want to be helpful. A well-worded "I" message can refuse the help tactfully, without embarrassing the other person: "Thank you for being so thoughtful, but today I think I can handle it myself. I'd like to be able to take you up on your offer another time, though!"

Responding to Others' Requests

Suppose, however, you are the one being asked to help someone. Often we need more information before we can respond to a request. Without enough information we often tend to say no. The example we just discussed about helping a person move is a good one. "Help me move" can mean anything from moving furniture up stairs to picking up the pizza for the hungry troops. It is important to understand what the *specific* request is before responding. *Asking for more information* or *paraphrasing* the request will often help clarify it. It's a good idea to begin with a phrase such as "Before I answer . . ."; this will hopefully prevent the person you are paraphrasing from feeling sure that you are going to say yes.

Once you know what the specific request is, if you decide to decline, it is important to *acknowledge the importance of the request* to the other person. In this way, the person will see that you are rejecting the *request*, rather than the *person*. Your turn-down should not be a put-down. "You know, that's a worthwhile project you're doing, but I think it's beyond my capabilities this week." Again, specifics are the key. Try to be clear about the conditions of your turn-down. Will you always turn down this request, or is it just that today or this week or right now is a problem?

Listening

Listening is probably the most important communication skill. Most of us are much better at talking than we are at listening. You need to actually listen to what the other person is *saying and feeling*. Most of us are already preparing a response instead of just listening.

There are several levels involved in being a good listener:

1. *Listen to the words and tone of voice, and observe body language.* Sometimes it is difficult to begin a conversation if there is a problem. There may be times when the words a person is saying don't tell you there is something bothering this person. Is the voice wavering? Does he or she appear to be struggling to find "the right words"? Do you notice body tension? Does he or she seem distracted? If you pick up on some of these signs, this person probably has more on his or her mind than words are expressing.

2. *Acknowledge having heard the other person.* Let the person know you heard him or her. This may be a simple "uh huh." Many times the only thing the other person wants is acknowledgment, or just someone to listen, because sometimes merely talking to a sympathetic listener is helpful.

3. *Acknowledge the content of the problem.* Let the other person know you understood the content and emotional level of the problem. You can do this by restating what you heard—for example, the content: "You are planning a trip." Or you can respond by acknowledging the emotions: "That must be difficult" or "You seem sad about it." When you respond on an emotional level, the results are often startling. These responses tend to open the gates for more expression of feelings and thoughts. Responding to either the content or emotion can also help communication along by discouraging the other person from repeating himself or herself.

4. *Respond by seeking more information.* This is especially important if you are not completely clear about what is being said or what is wanted. There is more than one useful method for seeking and getting information.

Getting More Information

Getting more information from another person is a bit of an art. Some of these methods are simple; others are more subtle.

Ask for More

Asking is the simplest way to get more information. "Tell me more" will probably get you more, as will "I don't understand . . . please explain," "I would like to know more about . . . ," "Would you say that another way?" "How do you mean?" "I'm not sure I got that," and "Could you expand on that?"

Paraphrase

Paraphrasing is a good tool if you want to make sure you understand what the other person meant (not just what he or she *said*). Paraphrasing can either help or hinder effective communication, though, depending on the way the paraphrase is worded. It is important to remember to paraphrase in the form of a *question,* not a statement:

Original statement:	"Well, I don't know. I'm really not feeling up to par. This party will be crowded, there'll probably be smokers there, and I really don't know the hosts very well, anyway."
(1) Paraphrased as a statement:	"Obviously, you're telling me you don't want to go to the party."
(2) Paraphrased as a question:	"Are you saying that you'd rather stay home than go to the party?"

The response to the first paraphrase might be anger: "No, I didn't say that! If you're going to be that way, I'll stay home for sure." Or the response might be no response—a total shutdown of communication, because of either anger or despair ("He just doesn't understand"). People don't like to be told what they meant.

The response to the second paraphrase might be more openness: "That's not what I meant. I'm just feeling a little nervous about meeting new people. I'd appreciate it if you'd stay near me during the party. I'd feel better about it and I might have a good time."

As you can see, the second paraphrase promotes further communication, and you have discovered the real reason the person was expressing doubt about the party. You have gotten more information from the second paraphrase (the question) and no new information from the first one (the statement).

Be Specific

If you want specific information, you must ask specific questions. We often automatically speak in generalities:

Doctor: How have you been feeling?

Patient: Not so good.

The doctor's question doesn't produce much in the way of information about the patient's condition. "Not so good" isn't very useful. Here's how the doctor gets more information:

Doctor: Are you still having those sharp pains in your left arm?

Patient: Yes. A lot.

Doctor: How often?

Patient: A couple of times a day.

Doctor: How long do they last?

Patient: A long time.

Doctor: About how many minutes, would you say?

And so on. Physicians have been trained in ways to get specific information from patients, but most of us have not been trained to ask specific questions. Again, simply *asking for specifics* often works: "Can you be more specific about . . . ?" "Are you thinking of something particular?" If you want to know "why," be specific about what it is. If you ask a specific question, you will be more likely to get a specific answer.

Simply asking *"Why?"* can unnecessarily prolong your attempt to get specific information. In addition to being a general rather than a specific word, *why* makes a person think in terms of cause and effect, and he or she may respond at an entirely different level than you had in mind. Most of us have experienced a three-year-old who just keeps asking "Why?" over and over and over again until the information he or she wants is finally obtained (or the parent runs from the room, screaming). The poor parent doesn't have the faintest idea what the child has in mind, and answers "Because . . ." in an increasingly specific order until the child's question is answered. Sometimes, however, the direction the answers take is entirely different from the subject of the child's question, and the child never gets the information he or she wanted. Rather than *why,* begin your questions with *who, which, when, where, or what.* These words promote a specific response. For example:

Doctor: I'm going to send you for a colonoscopy.

Patient: Why?

Words That Can Help or Hinder

Words That Help	*Words That Hinder*
• "I"	• "You"
• Right now, at this time, at this point, today	• Never, always, every time, constantly
• Who, which, where, when	• Obviously . . .
• How do you mean, please explain, tell me more, I don't understand	• Why

Doctor:	Well, because I feel that anyone with blood in his stool should have one.
Patient:	Why is that?
Doctor:	It's medically indicated.

And so on. This questioning could go on for a long time, and the patient's question "Why?" may hide any number of different concerns. Compare the conversation above with this one:

Doctor:	I'm going to send you for a colonoscopy.
Patient:	What do you think might be wrong?
Doctor:	I'm not sure. It's probably not serious, but you could have a cancer, such as lymphoma.
Patient:	Who does the colonoscopy? You?
Doctor:	No, Dr. Jones, the GI specialist, will do it.

And so on. Asking specific questions like these helps you communicate better and helps prevent misunderstandings.

Good communication skills help make life easier for everyone, especially when HIV/AIDS enters the picture. The skills discussed in this chapter will hopefully help smooth the communication process and bring you closer to your loved ones.

Suggested Reading

Beck, Aaron T. *Love Is Never Enough: How Couples Can Overcome Misunderstandings, Resolve Conflicts, and Solve Relationship Problems Through*

Cognitive Therapy. New York: Harper Collins, 1989. (A good introduction to cognitive techniques for couples.)

Burley-Allen, Madelyn. *Listening: The Forgotten Skill (A Self-Teaching Guide).* New York: John Wiley & Sons, 1995.

Fanning, Patrick, McKay, Matthew, and Davis, Martha. *Messages: The Communication Skills Book.* Oakland, Calif.: New Harbinger Publications, 1995.

McKay, Matthew, and Fanning, Patrick. *Couple Skills: Making Your Relationship Work.* Oakland, Calif: New Harbinger Publications, 1994.

14   Making Your Wishes Known: Advance Directives

All of us, whether ill or healthy, have feelings about our own death. Death may be feared, welcomed, accepted, or, all too often, pushed aside to be thought about at a different time. Somewhere, in the back of our minds, though, most of us have ideas about how and when we would like to die. For some of us, life is so important that we feel that everything should be done to sustain it. For others of us, life is important only so long as we can be active participants. For many people, the issue isn't really death but, rather, dying. We may have heard about the eighty-year-old who died skiing. This may be considered a "good" death. On the other hand, we may have a friend who died after spending a long time in a nursing home unaware of his or her surroundings. This is usually not what we would wish for ourselves.

Although none of us can have absolute control over his or her own death, this, like the rest of life, is something we can help manage. That is, we can express our wishes, make decisions, and probably add a great deal to the quality of our death. Proper management can lessen the negative impact of death on our survivors.

This chapter presents information that will help you better manage some of the legal issues of death, using legal documents called *advance directives*. As you read this chapter, bear in mind that each state has different laws about advance directives. You can get information and forms specific for your state by contacting Choice In Dying. The address is on page 209.

Living Will

The living will is probably the best known of the advance directives. It allows you to legally refuse life-support measures when you are considered to be near the end of your life—usually within six months.

The living will is widely available and serves a useful purpose. However, it is much less flexible than other advance directives, such as the durable power of attorney for health care. Remember, too, that the living will does not have legal standing in every state. Be sure to find out what your options are.

Durable Power of Attorney for Health Care

A durable power of attorney for health care (DPAHC) lets you do two things: (1) state your wishes about the kind of medical care you would like to receive, and (2) appoint an *agent* to make health care decisions for you when you cannot do so for yourself. A DPAHC, like a living will, can help protect you from "heroic" life-saving measures if you do not want them. However, the two documents have some important differences.

- A living will is good only in case of a terminal illness, whereas a DPAHC can apply to any illness.

- A living will enables you only to refuse treatment, whereas a DPAHC allows you to accept, refuse, or withdraw different forms of treatment.

- A living will does not allow you to appoint an agent. A DPAHC does.

In your DPAHC, you can include guidelines for your agent about what kind of health care you would like, under what circumstances. For example, you may indicate that you want everything possible done to keep you alive, no matter what your condition, or you may ask that you do not receive any treatment or food if you are in a coma or near death. Although you do not have to write down your wishes, doing so can be reassuring for family members and for doctors who see your DPAHC form.

Note that it is especially important to have a durable power of attorney for health care if you wish to choose your partner or someone who is not a blood relative as your agent. Otherwise, it's possible that your medical decisions will end up being made by a family member who may be unaware of or disagree with your wishes.

The agent named in your durable power of attorney for health care has the power to make medical decisions for you only when you are unable to make decisions yourself (for example, if you are in a coma or are taking medications that affect your alertness). The agent can make decisions only about your medical care, not about finances or other matters.

The durable power of attorney offers great flexibility and can be more useful than a living will. However, it may not have legal recognition in your state. Be sure to check.*

Creating a DPAHC means making many decisions. In the following section we'll cover each of the major issues that is likely to appear on your state's DPAHC form.

Choosing a Health Care Agent

Begin by deciding who you want as your agent. The person can be a friend or family member; it cannot be the physician who is providing your care. There are some considerations to be made in choosing your agent. First, the person should generally be available in the geographic area where you live. If the agent is not available to make decisions for you, he or she is not much help. Just to be on the safe side, you can also name a backup agent, who would act in your behalf if your first-choice agent were not available. Second, you must be sure that this person thinks like you think or at least is willing to carry out your wishes. Third, the person must be someone who you feel would be able to carry out your wishes. Sometimes a partner or child is not the best agent because this person is too close to you emotionally. For example, if you wish not to be resuscitated while in a severe coma, your agent has to be able to tell the doctor not to resuscitate. This decision could be difficult or impossible for a family member or partner to make on the spot. Be sure the person you choose as your agent is up to such a task. Finally, you want your agent to be someone who will not find this job to be too much of an emotional burden. Thus, the person has to be comfortable with the role, as well as willing and able to carry out your wishes.

In review, look for these characteristics in an agent:

- Someone who is likely to be available should he or she need to act on your behalf
- Someone who understands your wishes and is willing to carry them out
- Someone who is emotionally prepared and able to carry out your wishes

---

*Some states have other advance directives, besides living wills and DPAHCs, that we do not cover here.

- Someone who will not be emotionally burdened by carrying out your wishes

As you can see, finding the right agent is a very important task. You may want to talk to several people before making your choice; these may be the most important interviews that you ever conduct. We'll talk more about discussing your wishes with family, friends, and your doctor later.

Your Wishes Concerning Medical Treatment

The other major decision you'll need to make has to do with what kind of medical care you would like, under what circumstances. In other words, what are your directions to your agent? Some forms give you several statements to choose from, or leave a space in which you can write your own statement. Here are some sample statements:

> I do *not* want my life to be prolonged and I do *not* want life-sustaining treatment to be provided or continued: (1) if I am in an irreversible coma or persistent vegetative state; or (2) if I am terminally ill and the application of life-sustaining procedures would serve only to artificially delay the moment of my death; or (3) under any other circumstances where the burdens of the treatment outweigh the expected benefits. I want my agent to consider the relief of suffering and the quality as well as the extent or the possible extension of my life in making decisions concerning life-sustaining treatment.

> I want my life to be prolonged and I want life-sustaining treatment to be provided *unless I am in a coma or vegetative state* which my doctor reasonably believes to be irreversible. Once my doctor has reasonably concluded that I will remain unconscious for the rest of my life, I do *not* want life-sustaining treatment to be provided or continued.

> I want my life to be prolonged to the greatest extent possible without regard to my condition, the chances I have for recovery, or the cost of the procedures.

Some DPAHC forms simply make a "general statement of authority granted," in which you give your agent full power to make decisions. You do not write out the details of what these decisions should be; you are trusting your agent to follow your wishes. Since these wishes are not explicitly written, it is very important that you discuss them in detail with your agent.

Other Statements of Desires, Special Provisions, or Limitations

All forms also have a space in which you can write out any specific wishes that either limit or add to the authority you have given your agent. You are not required to give specific details but may wish to do so. Knowing what details to write is a little complicated because you do not know the exact circumstances in which the agent will have to act. However, you can get some idea by asking your doctor about what he or she thinks are the most likely things to happen to someone with your condition. Then you can direct your agent on how to act. Your specific directions can cover outcomes, specific circumstances, or both. If you discuss outcomes, the statement should focus on which types of outcomes would be acceptable and which would not—for example, "Resuscitate if I can continue to fully function mentally."

Following are two of the more common specific circumstances that are encountered with HIV/AIDS.

- *AIDS dementia complex* is a disease that can leave you with little or no mental function. In spite of this, it is generally not life threatening, at least not for a long time. However, things happen to people with AIDS dementia complex that can be life threatening, such as pneumonia, meningitis, and wasting. What you need to do is decide how much treatment you want. For example, do you want antibiotics if you get pneumonia? Do you want to be resuscitated if you die in your sleep? Would you like a feeding tube if you are unable to feed yourself? Remember, it is your choice as to how you answer each of these questions. You may not want to be resuscitated, but may want a feeding tube. You may want to use all means to sustain life or, more conservatively, you may not want any special means used to sustain life.

- You may have a *very bad lung function* that will not improve. Should you be unable to breathe on your own, do you want to be placed in an intensive care unit on mechanical ventilation (a breathing machine)? Remember, this is a situation in which you will not improve. To say that you never want ventilation is very different from saying that you don't want it if it is used to sustain life when no improvement is likely. Obviously, mechanical ventilation can be life saving in such crises as a severe asthma attack, when it is used for a short time until the body can regain its normal function. Here the issue is not whether to use mechanical ventilation ever, but rather when or under what circumstances you wish it to be used.

These examples may give you some ideas regarding the directions to give in your durable power of attorney for health care. Again, to better understand how to write such directions or how to make them more personal to your own condition, you might want to talk with your physician about what the common problems and decisions are for people like you.

In summary, there are several decisions you need to make in directing your agent on how to act in your behalf:

- Generally, *how much treatment do you want?* This can range from the very aggressive—that is, doing many things to sustain life—to the very conservative—doing almost nothing to sustain life, except to keep you clean and comfortable.

- Given the types of life-threatening things that are likely to happen to people with your condition, *what sorts of treatment do you want and under what conditions?*

- If you become *mentally incapacitated*, what sorts of treatment do you want for *other illnesses*, such as pneumonia?

Many people get this far. That is, they have thought through their wishes about dying and have even written them down in a DPAHC. This is an excellent beginning, but not the end of the job. A good manager has to do more than just write a memo. He or she has to see that the memo gets delivered. If you really want your wishes carried out, it is important that you share them fully with your agent, your family, and your doctor. This is often not an easy task. In the following pages, we will discuss ways to make these conversations easier.

Talking with Your Family, Friends, and Agent

Before you can discuss your wishes with family, friends, and agent, all interested parties need to have copies of your durable power of attorney for health care. Once you have completed the documents, have them notarized or witnessed and signed. Make several copies at any copy center. You will need copies for your agent, family members, and your doctor. You may also want to give one to your lawyer.

Now you are ready to talk about your wishes. Nobody likes to discuss his or her own death or that of a loved one. Therefore, it is not surprising that when you bring up this subject the response is often "Oh, don't think about that," or "That's a long time off," or "Don't be so morbid, you're not that sick." Unfortunately, this is usually enough to end the conversation. Your job as a self-manager is to keep the conversation open. Here are some suggestions on how to begin your discussion of this subject:

- *Prepare your durable power of attorney*, and then *give copies* to the appropriate family members or friends. *Ask them to read it* and then set a specific time to *discuss it*. If they give you one of those responses mentioned above, say that you understand that this is a difficult topic, but that it is important to you to discuss it with them. This is a good time to practice the "I" messages discussed in Chapter 13. For example, "I understand that death is a difficult thing to talk about. However, it is very important to me that we have this discussion."

- You might get *blank copies* of the DPAHC form for all your family members and suggest that *you all fill them out and share them*. Present this task as an important aspect of being a mature adult and family member. Making this a family project in which everyone is involved may make it easier to discuss. Besides, it will help to clarify everyone's values about the topics of death and dying.

- If these two suggestions seem too difficult or, for some reason, are impossible to carry out, you might *write a letter* or prepare an *audiotape* to send to members of your family. In the letter or tape, say why you feel your death is an important topic to discuss and that you want them to know your wishes. Then state your wishes, providing reasons for your choices. At the same time, send each person a copy of your DPAHC. Ask that they each respond in some way, or perhaps you can set aside some time to talk in person or on the phone.

Talking with Your Doctor

From our research we have learned that, in general, people have a much more difficult time talking to their doctors about their wishes surrounding death than to their families. In fact, only a very small percentage of people who have written DPAHCs ever share these with their physicians. There are several reasons why it is important that such a discussion take place. First, you need to *be sure that your doctor has values that are compatible with your wishes*. If you and your doctor do not have the same values, it may be difficult for him or her to carry out your wishes. Second, *your doctor needs to know what you want*. This allows him or her to take appropriate actions, such as writing orders to resuscitate or not to use mechanical resuscitation should this be needed. Third, *your doctor needs to know who your agent is and how to contact this person*. If an important decision has to be made and your wishes are to be followed, the doctor must talk with your agent. It is important to give your doctor a copy of your durable power of attorney for health care, so that it can become a permanent part of your medical record.

As surprising as it may seem, many physicians find it difficult to discuss death and how it might occur with their patients. After all, they are in the business of helping to keep people alive and well. They don't like to think about their patients dying. On the other hand, most doctors want their patients to have durable powers of attorney for health care. This relieves them of pressure and worry.

If you wish, *plan a time with your doctor when you can discuss your wishes*. This should not be a side conversation at the end of a regular visit. Rather, start a visit by saying, "I want a few minutes to discuss with you my wishes in the event of a serious problem or impending death." When you put it this way, most doctors will make time to talk with you. If the doctor says that he or she does not have enough time, then ask when you can make another appointment to talk about it. This is a situation in which you may need to be a little assertive. Sometimes a doctor, like your family members or friends, might say "Oh, you don't have to worry about that, let me do it," or "We'll worry about that when the time comes." Again, you will have to take the initiative, using an "I" message to communicate that this is important to you and that you do not want to put off the discussion.

Sometimes doctors do not want to worry you. They think they are doing you a favor by not describing all the unpleasant things that might happen to you, or the potential treatments, in the case of serious problems. You can help your doctor by telling him or her that having control and making some decisions about your future will ease your mind. Not knowing or not being clear on what will happen is more worrisome than being faced with the facts, unpleasant as they may be, and dealing with them.

Even if you are aware of all of the above, it is still sometimes hard to talk with your doctor. Therefore, it might also be helpful to *bring your agent with you* when you have this discussion. The agent can facilitate the discussion and, at the same time, meet your doctor. This way, everyone has a chance to clarify any misunderstandings about your wishes. It opens the lines of communication so that if your agent and physician have to act to carry out your wishes, they can do so with few problems.

So now you have done all the important things. You can rest easy. The hard work is over. However, remember that you can change your mind at any time. Your agent may no longer be available, or your wishes might change. Be sure to keep your durable power of attorney for health care updated. Like any legal document, it can be revoked or changed at any time.

One last note: Many states recognize durable powers of attorney for health care that are created in another state. However, this is not always the case. As of 2000, this is an unclear legal issue. To be on the safe side, if you move or spend a lot of time in another state, it is best to check with a lawyer in that state to see if your document is legally binding there.

Making your wishes known about how you want to be treated in case of serious or life-threatening illness is one of the most important tasks of self-management. The best way to do this is to prepare a DPAHC and share it with your family, close friends, and physician.

Be sure to check on the appropriate forms for your state by asking your doctor or lawyer or by writing to Choice In Dying (see below).

Resources

Making Your Wishes Known

Choice In Dying
475 Riverside Dr.
New York, NY 10015
1-800-989-9455
Web site: www.choices.org.

Suggested Reading

Cantor, Norman L. *Advance Directives and the Pursuit of Death with Dignity.* Bloomington: Indiana University Press, 1993.

King, Nancy M. P., *Making Sense of Advance Directives.* Washington D.C.: Georgetown University Press, 1996.

15   Planning for Now and the Future

This book is about living well with HIV/AIDS by taking charge of day-to-day problems and challenges and coming up with ways to solve them. Whether your problem is getting used to a new medicine, starting a new exercise routine, or dealing with the death of someone you love, the principles are the same. In this chapter we discuss some of the big questions people often have trouble thinking about. These questions tend to be about sensitive and sometimes unmentionable aspects of life: sex, grief, becoming dependent, money issues, and death. We touch on each of them and offer some suggestions that you may find useful.

The future can be frightening for people with HIV/AIDS. The most common way that people deal with their fear about the future is that they *don't* deal with it. People with illness often put off doing or thinking anything about the future, because they find it depressing or they feel that there's nothing they can do to make any difference. Of course, if you *think* that nothing you do will make a difference, then you probably won't do anything, and your prediction will come true. While there are many things to be concerned about—including loss of sex and intimacy, disability, loss of independence, money problems, and even death—there are also some ways to approach these issues that will help to keep you from feeling overwhelmed.

Does My Illness Mean an End to Sex and Intimacy?

Having HIV/AIDS should not redefine a person as an asexual being who's lost interest in sex. If anything, a person who has to face and adapt to changes caused by a chronic disease needs the love and comfort of close, intimate relationships perhaps more than ever. However, this aspect of life is often ignored, denied, or feared. For one thing, people with HIV/AIDS are rightly concerned about the risk that they will spread HIV to others. After all, even those who take potent "cocktail" HIV medications can still spread the disease. Learning to practice safer sex is necessary, but it's hard, and sometimes it seems easier just not to bother. Some people worry that the strenuousness of sex will make them weaker. Sometimes HIV/AIDS itself can lead to changes in hormone levels and decreased sex drive. People with breathing difficulties worry that sex is too strenuous and will bring on an attack of coughing and wheezing, or worse. Some people worry about starting new relationships, be they casual or more enduring. They struggle with whether or not to disclose their HIV status or wonder when the right time is to tell others.

One of the most subtle and devastating barriers to fulfilling sexuality is the damage that HIV/AIDS may cause to your self-image and self-esteem. You may believe you are physically unattractive as a result of your disease or medication side effects—for example, because of lipodystrophy, shortness of breath, weight loss, or a sense of not being really a whole, functioning being. This may cause you to avoid sexual situations, and you may "try not to think about it."

Attitude and communication are the keys to resuming the sexual aspect of your relationships. You must believe that sex is a necessary and rewarding part of your life, and you must communicate that to your partner.

As of this writing there are few instructional materials on sexuality specifically written for people with physical disabilities. There are, however, a number of very useful how-to guides in the bookstores for those wanting to enhance their sexual relationships. If you understand and appreciate your own needs and preferences, and those of your partner, you can use creativity in adapting the activities described in these guides to your own relationship. It is important to avoid any assumptions that there is only one "right way" to be sexually fulfilled.

Here are some ways to help you enhance sexual fulfillment:

- *Talk about your HIV status.* Your partner or potential partner needs to know, and the sooner you do it, the sooner you can move on to healthy, enjoyable safer sex practices.
- *Try to establish a calm and relaxed atmosphere.* Stressful or highly emotional conversations tend to cause anxiety and are not conducive to satisfying sexual activities.
- *Find activities and positions that are fun and comfortable for both of you.* Try to achieve open communication with your partner about what you like and want in the course of sexual activities.

- *Avoid sexual activity when you feel really tired.*
- *Avoid sexual activity right after a big meal.*
- *Avoid drinking alcohol before sex.*
- If you have trouble with sexual performance, *check with your doctor to see if you are taking medication that may be the cause.* Adjusting your dosage or switching to another medication may help.
- *Keep physically fit.* Being fit enhances sexual performance.
- *Get away to enjoy a romantic weekend.*
- *Consult a professional experienced in sexual counseling* if you are having chronic problems with arousal or a chronic loss of interest in sex. Short-term problems are often due to depression.

Grieving: A Normal Reaction to Bad News

When we experience any kind of a loss—small (such as losing a favorite possession) or large (such as losing a life partner or facing a disabling or terminal illness)—we go through an emotional process of grieving and coming to terms with the loss. A person with a chronic, disabling health problem experiences a variety of losses—loss of confidence, loss of self-esteem, loss of independence, loss of lifestyle, and perhaps the most painful of all, the loss of positive self-image if the condition has an effect on personal appearance.

Elisabeth Kübler-Ross, who has written extensively about this process, describes the following stages of grief:

- *Shock,* when we feel both a mental and a physical reaction to the initial recognition of the loss
- *Denial,* when we tell ourselves, "No, it can't be true," and proceed to act for a time as if it were not true
- *Anger,* when we ask, "Why me?" and search for someone or something to blame ("If the doctor had diagnosed it early enough, I'd have been cured," or "The job caused me too much stress.")
- *Bargaining,* when we say to ourselves, to someone else, or to God, "I'll never smoke again . . . ," or "I'll follow my treatment regimen absolutely to the letter . . . , "or "I'll go to church every Sunday . . ." ". . . if only I can get over this."

- *Depression,* when the real awareness sets in, we fully confront the truth about the situation, and experience deep feelings of sadness and hopelessness
- *Acceptance,* when we eventually recognize that we must deal with what has happened, and make up our minds to do what we have to do

We do not pass through these stages in a linear, out-of-one-and-into-the-next fashion. We are more apt to have several, or even many, flip-flops back and forth between them. Don't be discouraged if you find yourself angry or depressed again just when you thought you had reached acceptance. Many people get stuck at the anger and depression stages of the grief process; however, as we discussed in Chapter 8, there are several ways for you to move beyond these and toward acceptance.

What if I Can't Take Care of Myself Anymore?

Becoming helpless and dependent is the most basic fear among people who have potentially disabling health problems. This fear usually has physical as well as financial, social, and emotional components.

Physical Concerns of Day-to-Day Living

As your condition changes over time, you may need to consider changing your living situation. Change may involve hiring someone to help you in your home or moving to a living situation where help is provided. The decision about which alternative is best will be related to your needs and how they can best be met.

The first thing you will need to do is carefully *evaluate what you can do for yourself* and what activities of daily living will require some kind of help. These activities include the everyday things like getting out of bed, bathing, dressing, preparing and eating your meals, cleaning house, shopping, and paying bills. Most people can do all of these, even though they may have to do them more slowly, with some modification, or with some help from gadgets.

Some people, though, may eventually find that they are no longer able to do some of these activities without help from somebody else. For example, you may still be able to fix meals, but your mobility may be impaired to the degree that shopping is no longer possible. Or, if you have problems with fainting or sudden bouts of unconsciousness, you might need to have somebody around at all times.

When you have analyzed your situation, you should make a list, with one column for those activities that you need help with and another column for some ideas on what kind of help you might look for. For example:

Need Help With	*What Kind of Help to Look For*
Can't go shopping	• Get a friend to shop for me • Find a volunteer shopping service • Shop on the Internet or at a store that delivers • Ask a neighbor to shop for me when she does her own shopping • Get home-delivered meals
Can't be by myself	• Hire an around-the-clock attendant • Move in with a relative or friend • Get a "life-line" emergency response system • Move to a board-and-care home • Move into a shared-housing community or a group home for people with HIV/AIDS

When you have listed your problems and their possible solutions, select the solution that seems the most workable, acceptable, and least expensive for your needs.

The selection should depend upon your finances, family or other resources you can call on, and how well any of the potential solutions will in fact solve your problem. Sometimes one solution will be the answer for several problems. For instance, if you can't shop and can't be alone, and chores are reaching the point of a foreseeable need for help, you might consider that an assisted-living environment or group home will solve all these problems, since it offers assistance with meals, regular house cleaning, and transportation for errands and medical appointments.

Even if you are not of "retirement" age, many facilities accept younger people, depending on the facility's particular policies. Most facilities for the retired take residents as young as 50, or younger if one of a couple is the minimum age. If you are a young person, the local center for the disabled or independent living center should be able to direct you to an out-of-home care facility that is appropriate for you.

Your appraisal of your situation and needs may well be aided by sitting down with a trusted friend or relative and discussing your abilities and limitations. Sometimes another person can spot things that we ourselves overlook, or would like to ignore.

Make changes in your life slowly, incrementally. You don't need to change your whole life around to solve one problem. Remember, too, that you can always change your mind, if you don't "burn your bridges behind you." If you think that moving out of your own place to another living arrangement would be the thing to do, don't give up your present home until you are settled into your new home and are sure you want to stay there. If you think you need help with some activities, hiring help at home is less drastic than moving out, and may be enough for quite a while. If you can't be alone, and you live with a family member who is away during the day, maybe going to an adult or senior day care center will be enough to keep you safe and comfortable while your family is away. In fact, adult day care centers are ideal places to find new friends and activities geared to your abilities.

There are several kinds of professionals who can be of great help in giving you ideas about how to deal with your care needs:

- A *social worker* at your AIDS organization, center for the disabled, or hospital social services department can be very helpful with decisions about financial and living arrangement problems and with locating appropriate community resources. Some social workers are also trained in counseling the disabled in the area of emotional and relationship problems that may be associated with your health problem.

- A *licensed occupational therapist* can assess your daily living needs and suggest assistive devices or rearrangements in your environment to make life easier.

- An *attorney* should be on your "must see" list to help you set your financial affairs in order to preserve your assets, to prepare a proper will, and perhaps to execute a durable power of attorney for both health care and financial management. If finances are a concern, ask your local AIDS organization for the names of attorneys who offer free or low-cost services. Your local bar association or legal aid office can also refer you to a list of attorneys who are competent in this area.

Finding In-Home Help

If you find that you cannot manage your daily activities alone, your first option is usually to hire somebody to help. Most people just need a person called a *home aide,* or some similar title. Home aides provide no medically related services that require special licensing, but do help with bathing, dressing, meal preparation, and household chores.

You can find in-home help in a number of ways:

- *Home care agencies* are the easiest, but most expensive, way to find home care. You will usually find them listed under "home care" or "home nursing" in the telephone directory yellow pages. Such agencies are usually (but not always) private, for-profit businesses that supply caregiver staff to private individuals at home. The fees charged vary with the skill and license of the caregiver and will include an amount for Social Security, insurance, bonding, and profit for the agency. The fees are usually about double what you would expect to pay for someone you hire directly. The advantage, if you can afford it, is that the agency assumes all payroll responsibilities, including Social Security and federal and state taxes; responsibility for the skill and integrity of the attendant; and immediate replacement of an ill or no-show attendant. The agency pays the staff directly. The client has no involvement with paying the attendant, but pays the agency.

- *Registered nurses* (RNs) hired this way are very expensive, but it is rare for home care for a chronically ill person to require a registered nurse. *Licensed vocational nurses* (LVNs) will cost somewhat less, but are still expensive and are usually not needed unless there are nursing services required (such as dressing changes, injections, ventilator management, etc.). *Certified nursing assistants* (CNAs) have some basic training in nursing, are much less expensive, and can provide satisfactory care for any but the most critically ill person at home. Most agencies supply *home aides* as well as licensed staff. Unless you are bedridden or require some procedure that must be done by someone with a certain category of license, a home aide is probably the most appropriate for your needs.

- *Registries* supply prescreened lists of attendants or caregivers from which you select the one you wish to hire. You will be charged a placement fee, usually equal to one month's pay of the person hired. The agency will assume no liability for the skill or honesty of the people on its list, and you will need to check references and interview carefully, just as you would someone who comes from any other source. This type of resource can be found in the yellow pages under the same listing as "home nursing agencies" or under "registries." Some agencies provide both their own staff and registries of staff for you to select from.

- *Senior centers and centers serving the disabled population* may also provide home help. They often have listings of people who have called to say that they want work as a home attendant or who have put up a notice on a bulletin board there. These job seekers are not screened; you will need to interview them carefully and check their references before hiring someone.

- *The classified "employment wanted" section of your local newspaper* can also be a good resource for experienced home care attendants. Since their patients usually progress to a need for more or sometimes less care than home attendants can provide, their jobs are by nature temporary, and they often must look for new work. You can find a competent helper through the newspaper, but the advice to interview carefully is valid here, too.

- *Word of mouth* is probably your best source of help. Look for someone who has employed a person, or who knows of somebody who has worked for an acquaintance. Putting the word out through your family and social network may result in a jewel.

- *Home sharing* may be a solution if you have space and can offer a home to someone in exchange for help. This arrangement works best if you need help mainly with household and garden chores. However, some people may be willing to provide personal care, such as help with dressing and bathing and meal preparation. Some communities have agencies or government bureaus that help home sharers and home sharees locate each other.

Finding Out-of-Home Care

If getting the care you need just isn't possible in your own home, it may be time to think about moving someplace where you can be safe and comfortable. Here are some of the options to look into.

Residential Care Homes

Residential care homes, or *board-and-care homes,* are licensed by the state or county social services agency. They provide nonmedical care and supervision for persons who cannot live alone. These homes fall into two categories: large and small. The small ones have about six "residents," who live in a family-like setting in a neighborhood residence. The large ones have more residents, sometimes hundreds, who live in a boarding house or hotel-like setting. They take meals in a central dining room and have individual or shared rooms, with activities taking place in large common rooms.

In either type of facility, the services to the residents are the same—all meals, assistance with bathing and dressing as needed, laundry, housekeeping, transportation to medical appointments, supervision, and assistance with taking medications. In the larger facilities, there are usually professional activities directors. Residents of the larger facilities usually need to be more independent, since there is generally not as much personal attention as in the smaller homes.

These homes are licensed in most states for either "elderly" (over 62) or "adult" (under 62). The adult category is further divided into facilities for the mentally ill, mentally retarded, and physically disabled.

It is important when considering a residential care home to evaluate the nature of the persons who are already living there to make sure that you will fit in. For example, some of these facilities may cater to individuals who are mentally confused. If you are mentally clear, you would not find much companionship there. If everyone is hard of hearing, you might find conversation tiring.

Although all homes are by law required to provide wholesome meals, you should make sure the cuisine is to your liking and meets your dietary needs. If you need a vegetarian or diabetic diet, for instance, be sure the operator is willing to prepare your special meals.

The monthly fees for residential care homes vary, depending on whether they are spartan or luxurious. The most spartan facilities cost about the same as the SSI (Supplemental Security Income) benefit and will take SSI beneficiaries, billing the government directly. The more luxurious the home is with respect to furnishings, neighborhood, services, and so on, the greater the cost. Even the nicest of these will probably cost less than full-time, twenty-four-hour, seven-day at-home care.

Skilled Nursing Facilities

Sometimes called *nursing homes* or *convalescent hospitals, skilled nursing facilities* provide the most comprehensive care for severely ill or disabled people. If you have PCP or toxoplasmosis, you may need to be transferred from an acute hospital to a skilled nursing facility for a period of rehabilitation before going home.

No care situation seems to inspire more fear than the prospect of having to go to a nursing home. "Horror stories" in the news media help to foster the anxiety about what awful fate will befall anyone who has the misfortune to have to go to one. However, public scrutiny is valuable in helping to ensure that standards of care and humane and competent treatment are provided. It must be remembered that nursing homes serve a critical need. When you really need a nursing home, there is usually no other care situation that will meet your need.

Skilled nursing facilities provide medically related care for people who are no longer able to be in a nonmedical care situation. For example, you may need intravenous or injected medications that must be administered or monitored by professional nursing staff. Or you may be very physically limited, needing help with getting in and out of bed, eating, bathing, or dealing with bladder or bowel control. Skilled nursing facilities can also manage care of feeding tubes, respirators, and other high-tech care equipment. If you are only partially or temporarily disabled, you may need a skilled nursing facility for physical, occupational, or speech therapy; wound care; or other therapies.

Not all nursing homes provide all types of care. Some specialize in rehabilitation and therapies, and some specialize in long-term custodial care. Some provide high-tech nursing services; others do not.

In selecting a nursing home, you should seek the help of the *hospital discharge planner* or *social worker,* or a similar professional from a home care agency or center for the disabled. There are organizations that monitor local nursing homes. Each nursing home is required by law to post in a prominent place the name and phone number of the "ombudsman," the person assigned by the state licensing agency to assist patients and their families with problems in relation to their nursing home care. The agencies that can help you with this are listed in the yellow pages under "social service organizations."

Hospice

Although it isn't for everyone, hospice care is an important option that everyone should at least know about. Hospice philosophy is based on the belief that death is part of life and is something we will all experience. Therefore, hospice care concentrates on relieving pain and supporting emotional and spiritual needs. Hospice care doesn't emphasize prolonging life as long as is medically possible. Instead, the individual is given an environment to reflect on life and develop a sense of peace. The hope is that with good hospice care, a person can meet the end more peacefully than might otherwise be possible.

Many communities have excellent hospice facilities where people with serious illnesses can live and be cared for during the final stage of life. Hospice care can often be provided in your own home, too. The best way to find out about hospice care is through your local AIDS service organization or through your medical care site.

Will I Have Enough Money to Pay for My Care?

Next to the basic fear of physical dependency, the greatest fear of most people with serious illness is not having enough money to pay for their needs. Being sick often requires care and treatment that is expensive. If you are too ill or disabled to work, the loss of income and health insurance coverage may present an overwhelming financial burden. You can, however, avoid some of the risks by planning ahead and knowing your resources. There are a number of government benefit programs you should know about.

- *Social Security.* If you are too sick to work—either permanently or for some extended period—you may be entitled to draw Social Security on the basis of your disability. People with symptomatic HIV infection may be able to document their disability simply by showing that they have had one or more illnesses—such as *Pneumocystis* pneumonia (PCP), toxoplasmosis, or HIV wasting syndrome—that lead to "automatic" disability. People who haven't had one of these illnesses may have to get other documentation in order to qualify. If you qualify and have dependent children, they would also receive Social Security benefits. If you have been disabled for a specified period (as of this writing, two years) you may be entitled to Medicare coverage for your medical treatment needs.

- *Medicaid and SSI.* If you have only minimal savings and little or no income, the federal Medicaid program can pay for medical treatment and long-term skilled or custodial care. The eligibility rules on assets and income differ from state to state. If you have savings of less than the U.S. median of one month's wages, and income at or slightly above the official federal "poverty line" (this changes from year to year), you should consult your local social services department to see if you are entitled to benefits. If Social Security benefits are unavailable or insufficient, the Supplemental Security Income (SSI) program is available to those who meet the same eligibility criteria as for Medicaid.

If you have some savings, you will have to pay for your care until you have "spent down" to meet the asset limitation criteria for Medicaid and SSI. If you have income above a certain level, you will be responsible for what is termed a "co-payment," or "share-of-cost," which you must pay before Medicaid will begin to supplement.

The social work department in the hospital where you have obtained treatment can advise you about your own situation and your eligibility for these programs. The local agency serving the disabled also usually has benefits counselors or advisors who can refer you to programs and resources for which you may be eligible. Local AIDS and community service organizations often have benefits counselors who are knowledgeable about the ins and outs of health care insurance.

Be warned: Although the government can provide a helpful (and in some cases life-saving) safety net, dealing with government agencies is difficult. Be patient, expect problems, and keep at it.

I Need Help, but I Don't Want Help— Now What?

We all emerge from childhood reaching for and cherishing every possible form of independence—the driver's license, the first job, the first checking account, the first time we go out and don't have to tell anyone where we're going or when we'll be back, and so on. In these and many other ways, we demonstrate to ourselves as well as to others that we are in charge of our lives and able to take care of ourselves without any help from parents.

If a time comes when we must face the realization that we need help, that we can no longer manage completely on our own, it may seem like we are making a return to childhood and having to let somebody else be in charge of our lives. This dependency can be very painful and embarrassing. Some people in this situation become depressed and can no longer find any joy in life. Others fight off the recognition of their need for help, thus placing themselves in possible danger and making life difficult and frustrating for those who would like to be helpful. Some people give up completely and expect others to take total responsibility for their lives, demanding attention and services from their partners, friends, and family. If you are having one or more of these reactions, you can help yourself feel better and develop a more positive response.

"Let me have the courage to change the things I can change, the serenity to accept the things I cannot change, and the wisdom to know the difference." This concept is fundamental to staying in charge of your life. You must be able to correctly evaluate your situation. You must identify those activities that require the help of somebody else (going shopping or cleaning house, for instance) and those activities you can still do on your own (getting dressed, paying bills, writing letters). This means making decisions, and as long as you keep the decision-making prerogative, you are in charge. It is important to make a decision and take action while you are still able to do so, before circumstances intervene and the decision gets made for you. That means being realistic and honest with yourself.

There are several approaches you can take to get help and still stay in charge of your life:

- *Talk with a sympathetic listener,* either a professional counselor or a sensible, close friend or family member. An objective listener often helps by pointing out alternatives and options that you may have overlooked or were not aware of. Such a person can provide information or another point of view or interpretation of a situation that you would not have come upon yourself. This is part of the self-management process. Be very careful, however, in evaluating advice from someone who has something to sell you. There are many people whose solution to your problem just happens to be whatever it is they are selling—health or burial insurance policies, special furniture, "sunshine cruises," special magazines, or health foods with curative properties.

- *Be as open and reasonable as you can be* when talking with family members or friends who offer to be helpful, yet at the same time try to make them understand that you will reserve for yourself the right to decide how much and what kind of help you will accept. They will probably be more cooperative and understanding if you say, "Yes, I do need some help with . . . , but I still want to do . . . myself."

- *Insist on being consulted.* Lay the ground rules with your helpers early on. Ask to be presented with choices, so that you can decide what is best for you as you see it. If you try to objectively weigh the suggestions made to you and don't dismiss every option out of hand, people will consider you able to make reasonable decisions and will continue to provide you the opportunity to do so.

- *Be appreciative.* Recognize the goodwill and the efforts of those who want to help. Even though you may be embarrassed, you will maintain your dignity by accepting with grace the help that is offered, if you need it. If you are truly convinced that you are being offered help you don't need, you can decline it with tact and appreciation. For example, you can say, "I appreciate your offer to have Thanksgiving dinner at your house, but I'd like to continue having it here. I could really use some help, though—maybe with the clean-up after dinner."

- *Consult a professional counselor* if you are at length unable to come to terms with your increasing need to be dependent on others for help in managing your living situation. This should be someone who has experience with the emotional and social issues of people with disabling health problems. Your local agency for providing services to the disabled should be able to refer you to the right kind of counselor. The local or national organization dedicated to serving people with HIV/AIDS can also refer you to support groups and classes to help you in dealing with your condition. You should be able to locate the agency you need through the telephone book yellow pages under the listing "social service organizations."

We need to be sure that we do reach out to family and friends and ask for the help we need when we recognize that we can't go on alone. It sometimes happens that, expecting rejection, people fail to ask for help. Some people try to hide their need in fear that their need will cause loved ones to withdraw. Families often complain, "If we'd only known . . ." when it is revealed that a loved one had needs for help that were unmet.

If you really cannot turn to close family or friends because they are unable or unwilling to become involved in your care, there are agencies dedicated to providing for such situations. Through your local social service department's "adult protective services" program or family services association, you should be able to locate a "case manager" who will be able to organize the resources in your community to provide the help you need. The social services department in your local hospital can also put you in touch with the right agency.

I'm Afraid of Death

Fear of death is something most of us begin to experience only when something happens to bring us face-to-face with the possibility of our own death. Losing someone close, surviving an accident that could have been fatal, or learning about a health condition that may shorten life usually causes us to consider the inevitability of our own passing. Many people, even then, try to avoid facing the future because they are afraid to think about it.

If you are ready to think about your own future—about the imminent or distant prospect that your life will most certainly end—then the ideas that follow will be useful to you. If you are not ready to think about it just yet, put this section aside and come back to it later.

Getting Your House in Order

The most useful way to come to terms with your eventual death is to take positive steps to prepare for it. This means "getting your house in order" by attending to all the small and large details that are necessary. If you continue to avoid dealing with these details, you will create problems for yourself and for those who will become involved with your situation in a significant way. There are several components to getting your house in order:

- *Decide and then convey to others your wishes about how and where you want to be during your last days and hours.* Do you want to be in a hospital or at home? When do you want life-prolonging procedures stopped? At what point do you want to let nature take its course when it is determined that death is inevitable? Who should be with you—only the few people who are nearest and dearest, or all the people you care about and want to see one last time?

- *Make a will.* Even if your estate is a small one, you may have definite preferences about who should have what. If you have a large estate, the tax implications of a proper will may be very significant.

- *Make arrangements, or at least plans, for your funeral.* Your grieving family will be very relieved not to have to decide what you would want and how much to spend. There are prepaid "future need" funeral plans available, and you can purchase burial space of the type you prefer.

- *Prepare an advance directive* (see Chapter 14) and also a durable power of attorney that will let someone manage your financial affairs. You should discuss your health care wishes with your personal physician, even if he or she doesn't seem to be very interested. (Your physician may also have trouble facing the prospect of losing you.) Be sure to include some kind of document or notation in your medical records that indicates your wishes in case you can't communicate them when the time comes.

- *Be sure that the persons you want to have handle things after your death are aware of all that they need to know*—your wishes, your plans and arrangements, and the location of necessary documents. You will need to talk to them, or at least prepare a detailed letter of instructions and give it to someone who can be counted on to deliver it to the proper person when necessary. You may not want your spouse or partner to have to take on such things as funeral responsibilities, but he or she may be the best person to keep your letter and to know when to give it to your designated agent. You can purchase at any well-stocked stationery store a preorganized kit in which you place a copy of your will, your durable power of attorney, important papers, and information about your financial and personal affairs. The kit also contains forms that you fill out about bank and charge accounts, insurance policies, the location of important documents, your safe-deposit box and where the key is kept, and so on. This is a handy, concise way of getting everything together that anyone might need to know about.

- *"Finish business" with the world around you.* Mend your relationships. Pay your debts, both financial and personal. Say what needs to be said to those who need to hear it. Do what needs to be done. Forgive yourself. Forgive others.

- *Share your feelings about your death.* Most family and close friends are reluctant to initiate such a conversation but appreciate it if you bring it up. You may find that there is much to say to and to hear from your loved ones. If you find that they are unwilling to listen to you talk about your death, find someone who will be comfortable and empathic in listening to you. Your partner, family, and friends may be able to listen to you later on. Remember, those who love you will also go through the stages of grieving when they have to think about the prospect of losing you.

Dying

A large component in the fear of death is fear of the unknown. "What will it be like?" "Will it be painful?" "What will happen to me after I die?"

Most people who die of a disease are ready to die when the time comes. Painkillers and the disease process itself weaken the body and mind, and the awareness of self diminishes without the realization that this is happening. Most people just "slip away," with the transition between the state of living and that of no longer living hardly identifiable. Reports from people who have been "brought back to life" after being in a state of "clinical death" indicate that they experienced a sense of peacefulness and clarity and were not frightened.

However, a dying person may sometimes feel very lonely and abandoned. Regrettably, many people cannot deal with their own emotions when they are around a person they know to be dying and so deliberately avoid that person's company, or they may engage in superficial chitchat, broken by long awkward silences. This is often puzzling and hurtful to the dying person, who needs companionship and solace.

You can help by telling your partner, family, and friends what you want and need from them—attention, entertainment, comfort, practical help, and so on. Again, when people have something positive to do, they are more able to cope with their emotions. If you can engage your loved ones in specific activities, they can feel needed and can relate to you around the activity. This will give you something to talk about, occupy time, or at least provide a definition of the situation for them and for you.

Again, if you choose to die at home, a *hospice* can be very helpful. Hospice organizations provide both physical and emotional care for people who are dying, as well as for their families.

Suggested Reading

Callanan, Maggie, and Kelley, Patricia. *Final Gifts: Understanding the Special Awareness, Needs, and Communications of the Dying.* New York: Bantam Books, 1997.

Carroll, David. *Living with Dying: A Loving Guide for Family and Close Friends.* New York: Shooting Star Press, 1991.

Kübler-Ross, Elisabeth. *Living with Death and Dying*. Indianapolis: Macmillan, 1997.

Leslie, Mark. *Dying with AIDS: Living with AIDS*. Muses Co., 1993.

Longaker, Christine. *Facing Death and Finding Hope: A Guide to the Emotional and Spiritual Care of the Dying*. New York: Doubleday, 1998.

16

Finding Resources

Amajor part of becoming a self-manager of your HIV/AIDS is knowing when you need help and how to find help. Seeking help to perform daily tasks and chores or to assist with other areas of your life does *not* mean that you have fallen victim to your illness. Rather, knowing where to go for help in specific areas of your life takes initiative—evaluation of your condition and your own capabilities. By becoming more aware of the symptoms you experience throughout the day, you can better predict the amount of energy and patience you will have to accomplish tasks. If you find that you come up short on energy, time, patience, or capability for some tasks, you can evaluate where help from other resources will preserve your own resources for those things most important to you.

The first resource you will probably go to for help is *family* or *close friends*. Some find it difficult, however, to ask for help from people they know. Finding the right words to ask for help is discussed in Chapter 13, "Communicating." Unfortunately, some people either do not have family or close friends to call on or cannot bring themselves to ask. If this is the case, you must look for other resources in your community. This chapter will show you how to search for resources and lists some of the most useful sources for the kind of help and information commonly needed by people with HIV/AIDS.

Getting Started: Finding Clues and Networking

Finding resources in your community is a little like a treasure hunt: creative thinking wins the game. Finding what you need may be as simple as looking in the telephone book and making a couple of phone calls. Other times, you will need to follow clues, including starting over when the clue leads to a dead end.

Where do you start? Suppose you find it difficult to prepare meals because prolonged standing is too tiring or painful. After some thought, you decide that you want to continue cooking for yourself rather than have someone else cook your meals. The next step, then, is to explore the prospect of having your kitchen altered so you can prepare meals from a seated position. Where can you find an architect or contractor who has knowledge of and experience in kitchen alterations for people with physical limitations? Looking at the yellow pages and the classified section of the newspaper reveals pages of ads and listings for architects and contractors; some say they specialize in kitchens, while others don't mention any specialty. None mentions anything about designing for physical limitations. A couple of phone calls to contractors listing kitchens as a specialty are unsuccessful in finding anyone experienced in kitchens for the physically limited.

Now what? You could call everyone listed until you find what you need. Not only would this be time consuming, but you may not feel comfortable about hiring the contractor you find until you talk to someone else who knows this person's work. Here is where creative thought and networking enter the picture. Who else do you know that might have information of this kind? Maybe someone who works with physically disabled people would have ideas—an occupational or physical therapist, an orthopedic supply store, your city or county's human services department or commission, the nearest independent living center for the disabled, the community college disabled services office, or your local AIDS service organization. You may talk to someone who doesn't have the answer but says, "Gosh, Jack So-and-So just had his kitchen remodeled to accommodate his wheelchair. Maybe he can help you find someone." Jack is probably a great lead to follow. He may be able to give you not only the name of someone who can do the work, but also some ideas about cost and other concerns before you go any further in the process. He's probably done much of the groundwork already and can save you time and trouble.

Suppose, however, that your search still isn't successful. Every community has people who are natural resources. These "naturals" seem to know everyone and know where everything is. They tend to be folks who have lived in the community a long time and have been involved in it. They are natural problem solvers—the ones people always seek out for advice. If you were to call such a person, he or she would probably know the answer or could set you on the right path to get the answer. The "natural" could be a friend, a business associate, the mail carrier, your physician, your pet's veterinarian, the checker at the corner grocery, the pharmacist, the bus or taxi driver, your child's school secretary, a real estate agent, the chamber of commerce receptionist, or the librarian. All you need to do is think of this person as an information resource.

Resources for Resources

Most searches for information begin with a single step and expand into a web of networking that will bring you into contact with unexpected resources.

The following list will give you many starting points for finding the resources you need.

- *The telephone book* is where most people start to look for community resources. Particularly if you need to hire someone to do something for you, the telephone book is full of people and organizations ready to help you.

- *Local AIDS information and referral services* are listed in your telephone book. Look under "AIDS information and referral," "United Way information and referral," or simply "information and referral" in your county or city government listings. Once you have an information and referral telephone number, your searches become much easier. These services maintain a huge file of referral addresses and telephone numbers for just about any kind of help you might need. Even if they don't have the answer to your need, they will almost always be able to refer you to another agency that can speed you along in your search.

- *Voluntary agencies dedicated to your disease* are one of the most important resources you can find for either information or help. For people with HIV/AIDS, this means your local AIDS foundation. Agencies of this type are funded by contributions from individuals and corporate sponsors and provide up-to-date information about your disease as well as support and direct services to people with AIDS. For a small membership fee, you can become a member of these organizations, which entitles you to receive regular bulletins by mail. You do not, however, have to be a member to qualify for their services. They are here to serve you.

- *National HIV/AIDS organizations* maintain telephone hotlines to offer information about all kinds of resources, many of which may be available in your community.

- *HIV/AIDS resource guides* are often published by local HIV/AIDS organizations and provide information about services and resources available to people with HIV/AIDS. The listings are categorized by type—financial, medical, social, and mental health and support—and are updated regularly.

- *Other community organizations, such as community centers and religious social service agencies,* also offer information and referral services as well as direct services. The latter may include classes, recreational opportunities, nutrition programs, legal and tax help, and social programs. There is probably a community center close to you. Your city government office or local librarian will know where they are, and the calendar section of your newspaper will usually have information about programs these organizations offer.

- *Religious groups* usually offer information and social services to those in need, either directly through the local church or synagogue or through the Council of Churches, Catholic Charities, or Jewish social service groups. To get help from religious organizations, start with your local church or synagogue; they will help you or refer you to someone who can help. You need not be a member of the religion or of its local organization to receive help.

- *Hospital and health care organizations* may also offer services. Many clinics caring for people with HIV/AIDS have access to excellent social workers and case managers who can give you much help. Call your local hospital, clinic, or health insurance plan and ask for their social service department. *Your doctor* will also be aware of the services available in the health care organizations he or she is affiliated with.

- *Libraries* are invaluable resources, particularly when you are looking for information about your disease. The library, and the *reference librarian* in particular, can serve as an information and referral service as well. Often the reference section of the library has a gem of a book or pamphlet that will give you listings of the resources you are looking for. The reference librarian can probably take you right to it—and perhaps show you others as well. Even if you think you are good at library research, it's a good idea to ask the reference librarian if you have overlooked something. Reference librarians see volumes of material cross their desks and are knowledgeable about community resources.

    If you don't have a computer, libraries often provide Internet access to the rapidly growing information and rescource organizations on the Web.

- *University and college libraries* are also open to the public. By law, in fact, the regional *government documents* sections of these libraries must be open to the public at no charge. Government publications exist on just about any subject, and the health-related publications are particularly extensive. You can find information on everything from organic gardening to detailed nutritional recipes. The librarians are usually very helpful, and these publications are "your tax dollars at work."

- *Medical school libraries,* if you are fortunate enough to have one in your community, are another resource for information (although they are not a place to look for help with tasks). Naturally, you would expect to find a great deal of information about disease and treatment at a medical library, but unless you have some special knowledge about medicine, the information you find there can be intimidating and confusing. Use medical libraries with care.

- *Backs of books* are another great resource. Look for the reading list (sometimes titled "Bibliography") and other resource lists at the back of a book related to your disease. Sometimes this information is easy to miss because it is found just before or after the index. Backs of books are helpful for finding information as well as names and addresses of agencies and other organizations.

- *Local newspapers* are an excellent source of information. The health or science editor and the calendar of events editor can also be very knowledgeable about community resources. Gay community newspapers in particular contain a great deal of information. Two newspaper sections that can be most helpful in your search for resources are the *calendar of events section* and the *classified section.* Organizations advertise classes, lectures, and other events in both of these sections. In the classifieds, look under "Announcements," "Health," or any other heading that looks promising (you'll find an index of the headings used by your newspaper printed at the front of the classified section). Even if you are not interested in the particular events advertised, the contact telephone numbers may be good leads in your search for something else. Look in other logical places for news stories that might be of interest, such as the pages around the calendar section or the health-and-fitness section (you might find an exercise program for people with your health problem there, for example).

- *The Internet* is an almost endless source of information about HIV/AIDS. Of course, you must have access to a computer at home, at work, or at the library that is connected to the Internet (either by modem or directly linked), and you have to be comfortable using the computer. But if you can solve these problems, the Internet can be a way to look up treatment options, ask questions, find out about studies—all kinds of information. The great thing about the Internet is that literally everything is there. The not-so-great thing about the Internet is that . . . literally everything is there. Anyone can put anything they want on the Internet. There's no one editing the material. The quality can vary drastically.

So how does one separate what's valid from what's not valid (or even crazy)? It can be hard to tell. On the World Wide Web, sites created by official organizations (such as the CDC, universities, or the major AIDS organizations) are reliable, and they generally have material that's in the mainstream of thought about AIDS. Information from newsgroups or "personal" web sites is often more interesting, but you may need to treat much of it skeptically. People may try to sell you things—look out for extravagant claims about new "cures." Discuss things you've heard about on the Internet with others. If something sounds too good to be true, it probably is.

All of these resources are just first steps. Once you've started down any path, you'll find that, with persistence and creativity, your information and support network will grow to give you many choices. You are not alone.

A Reference Guide to Key HIV/AIDS Resources

National Hotlines

National AIDS Hotline   (800) 342-2437
                                                          TTY (800) 243-7889

Operated by the Centers for Disease Control (CDC). Open 24 hours a day. Offers information, referrals to agencies, and trained counselors.

National Prevention Information Network (NPIN)   (800) 458-5231
                                                       TTY (800) 243-7012
                                                   e-mail: info@cdcnpin.org
                                                   Internet: www.cdcnpin.org

Provides access to all of the CDC's published information. You can get referrals to AIDS organizations and services, order publications, get information about

AIDS in the workplace, find out about the latest clinical trials, or use an automated service to get information via fax or e-mail. You can also order a free catalogue of HIV/AIDS education and prevention materials.

Internet Links

Things change quickly in the fields serving the HIV/AIDS community. Probably the most up-to-date information resources for people with HIV/AIDS are on the Internet. Here are four web sites that are excellent gateways to HIV/AIDS resources. Each has extensive links to more specific organizations and other resources.

HIVInSite (University of California, San Francisco)	http://hivinsite.ucsf.edu
Johns Hopkins AIDS Service	http://www.hopkins-AIDS.edu
The Body	http://www.thebody.com
AEGiS (Sisters of St. Elizabeth of Hungary—updated hourly)	http://www.aegis.com

For information on pharmaceutical patient-assistance programs, with a search engine to find specific drugs:

Association for Clinicians
for the Underserved   http://www.clinicians.org/pharmadoc.html
National Office
501 Darby Creek Road, Suite 20
Lexington, KY 40509-1606
Tel: (606) 263-0046
Fax: (606) 263-7580

e-mail: acu@clinicians.org

Index

Notes